Published by: Matt Bennett April 2022

Matt@Myrawintuition.com www.Myrawintuition.com

DISCLAIMER

The information and recipes contained within this book are neither intended to treat, cure, or diagnose any disease or illness, nor meant to replace your healthcare professional or family physician's advice. The techniques and advice described in this book represent the opinions of the author based on his experience. The author expressly disclaims any responsibility for any liability, loss or risk, personal or otherwise, which is incurred as a result of using any of the techniques, recipes, or recommendations suggested herein. If in any doubt, or if requiring medical advice, please contact the appropriate health professional.

Table of Contents

Introduction

Life is an ocean of inevitable change and your actions are the sails to your ship. It is your ability to control the direction of your actions that will determine the type of change you sail through in life. - Matt Bennett

Welcome to The 21-Day Raw Transformation Program, where you will learn how to successfully adopt a raw vegan diet in a healthy and sustainable way. This program is strategically designed with tools and resources to guide you through the transformation of your diet and lifestyle using a personalized approach that supports your unique circumstances.

Some of what you will learn:

• The five pillars of transforming your body, mind, and spirit
• How to reprogram the subconscious mind to support your goals
• How to set effective dietary boundaries that support your long-term success
• How to eliminate cravings on a raw vegan diet
• How to build a healthy relationship with food

This program also includes a 21-day raw vegan meal plan to show you how easy and delicious raw vegan eating can be!

The 3P Philosophy

People ask me how I have managed to eat a raw vegan diet for so many years while working a 9-5 job in the cold winters of Minnesota. They often guess I must have super-human willpower or that I am simply a freak of nature, but the truth is **anyone can do it**, with or without supernatural abilities.

The key is to change your frame of reference and understand that changing any aspect of a lifestyle can seem difficult at first, but the more you do something, *the easier it becomes* as time goes on.

I have found three core reasons that some people have trouble finding long-term success on a raw vegan diet: the lack of patience, practicality, and perseverance needed to maintain their new habits long enough that they become an easy and natural part of their routine.

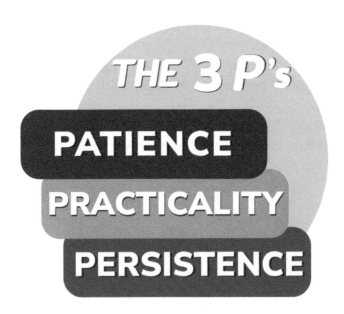

Patience

Any time we accept the challenge of learning something new, there will always be a period of time at the beginning where it feels difficult or frustrating. Though, over time, as we continue to practice and gain more experience, what once seemed difficult, gradually becomes more and more natural to us. This is why it is so important to be patient with yourself as you are starting to implement the concepts in this book – it truly takes time for these new habits to take root in your lifestyle. In addition, if you are used to eating a low fiber diet, it is even more important to take things slow to allow your gut microbiome time to adjust to higher levels of fiber.

One of the common themes I see with people that give up on this lifestyle is being in too much of a hurry to reach the end goal. There is nothing wrong with striving for maximum efficiency but sometimes being fixated on making giant leaps rather than progressing step-by-step can lead one to become burnt-out and discouraged. It took me roughly one year of progressively transitioning into the raw diet before I felt like I had developed a solid sense of the "how" and "why" behind making this lifestyle work for me. Even still today, entering my eleventh year of eating this way, I continue to evolve as I learn new things and tweak my diet and lifestyle as I find necessary. How I eat depends mainly on the selection of available produce at any given time. Each new season offers exciting and delicious foods to enjoy – flow with the seasons and stay flexible.

It can be helpful to think of this learning process as a marathon, not a sprint. You would not want to start a marathon running at full speed, or you would never finish the race – at least not with your best time. Begin running at a moderate pace that you can sustain for the duration of the race and along the way you can speed up or slow down as needed. You may stumble along the way (maybe by eating something that was not on your plan), which is perfectly fine – this is where having patience can make or break you – pick yourself up, regain your balance, and continue toward your goal. Never shame yourself if you stumble – have self-compassion, understand it is part of the learning and growing process, and appreciate the lesson of the experience.

This is your marathon, and you are running a course that is specific to you. Your life, circumstances, and needs are unique to you – do not compare yourself to anyone else's pace or results. Do not feel pressured, rushed, or responsible to live up to anyone's expectations of your results, other than your own. Keep in mind, that does not mean you should never push yourself outside of what makes you comfortable. Important growth and development happen when we are challenged, so it is essential to try new things and build an understanding of what works through trial and error. Always carry the intention that you will strive to do your best in every situation and even though you may stumble, you will be successful.

Practicality

I know how exciting it is to come across new information that deep down you know could be a game changer in your life and you want to do everything perfectly from the beginning. That is completely natural and there are a lot of inspiring raw food teachers out there that appear to have it all figured out. Though, the information they share (including my own) is the culmination of many years of trial and error and it is within those errors that the true education happens. I encourage you to set your goals and expectations high but be practical with regard to what it will take to get there.

I see all too often, someone living in a place like Minnesota trying to replicate, verbatim, the diet and lifestyle of someone in Costa Rica and becoming frustrated in the process, causing them to give up – not realizing they could have made a few simple adjustments to personalize this lifestyle in a way that is more appropriate for their situation. The overwhelming majority of people that I have seen struggle to maintain a plant-based diet do not take an approach that is practical for their circumstances and they burn out from preventable causes. Being practical means to be flexible and realistic with your mindset and the action steps you put in place to achieve your health and lifestyle aspirations.

If you live in a temperate climate, do not expect to have access to the same selection of fruits as someone living in the tropics. Even within the same state, the selection of fruits and vegetables can vary greatly, depending on the size of the city you live in. So, you will have to survey your local area and determine which produce you have access to throughout the year and then adapt your diet accordingly. The good news is that more and more cities are expanding their selection of fresh produce as the demand for healthy food continues to increase. More grocery stores are carrying organic options and local farmers markets are becoming extremely popular all over the world. So, even if you do not live in the tropics, that does not mean a raw vegan diet is unachievable – you just need to design it in a way that is practical for your situation.

Persistence

Most things worth doing will test your determination. I have never seen anyone accomplish their high-level goals by taking the path of least resistance. Just as the flavor of a tomato grown in a comfortable, temperature-controlled greenhouse is dull and bland compared to the full, vibrant flavors of a

tomato grown outdoors in the challenging elements –
overcoming something that challenges you will add flavor
and richness to your life. If you are serious about achieving
your health goals, you must be committed to your plan,
especially under stress when you are tempted to fall back into
old, familiar habits. That said, if you happen to fall off the
plan and give in to temptation (no matter how many times),
show yourself compassion, learn from the experience, and get
back on track with enthusiasm!

If, after reading this book, you believe the raw vegan way of
life holds the answers you seek, your level of persistence will
be a direct reflection of how dedicated you are to your own
health and happiness. We either make it happen or we make
excuses – the choice is yours. There are plenty of people out
there who say they want to achieve something but repeatedly
self-sabotage their progress and use their struggles as an
excuse to settle or give up – never allowing themselves to
experience the happiness and fulfillment they were entirely
capable of attaining – I do not think you are one of those
people.

The 21-Day Raw Transformation Program has all the tools
you need to confidently move beyond your comfort zone
without feeling overwhelmed. The most important tool you
have is your mind, and by embracing a positive mentality you
will change your behavior and how you speak to yourself –
making it easier to stay patient, practical, and persistent
towards any goal you want to achieve. Utilizing the three P's
creates a positive feedback loop that exponentially builds
your confidence and abilities the longer you practice them.

My Transition To A Raw Vegan Diet

My personal awakening to the raw vegan lifestyle began in 2011 after three major shifts in my consciousness. The first shift happened after a 10-day fruit and vegetable juice fast. I had been suffering from asthma, eczema, acne, low energy, poor sleep, brain fog, toxic thinking, colds, flus, congestion, constipation, and so much more.

After hearing about the health benefits of juicing and juice fasting, I gave it a try and immediately felt an improvement in my energy, sleep, and mental clarity. After a few days, I could not believe how much cleaner my airways felt. I was less congested and the asthmatic wheezing in my chest was noticeably improved.

By the tenth and final day of my juice fast, I had lost several pounds of extra weight that I was not even aware I had been holding on to - but more importantly, I had lost my illusions of what was required to be healthy. My whole life I was led to believe that I needed protein from meat and calcium from dairy products.

However, experiencing the way that I felt physically, mentally, and spiritually while juicing changed how I looked at food forever. I had felt something that I could not un-feel and so began my journey to discover the truth about health. I found myself immersed in health books, incessantly researching on the internet, and watching all the documentaries I could find.

This insatiable desire to understand why I felt so much better eating more plants and less animal foods led me to the teachings of Dr. Robert Morse N.D., who served me my second major shift in consciousness. He explained that every animal in nature had a species specific diet which perfectly aligned with their biological design. He went on to describe the four classifications of vertebrates:

Carnivore
Includes: Cats, lions, tigers, etc.
Diet: Meats, some vegetables, grass, herbs
Digestive System: Large mouth opening, unidirectional jaw (up and down only), large canine teeth, rough tongue, less than or equal to 1 pH with food in stomach, smooth and short small intestine – 3 to 6 times body length, short and smooth non-sacculated colon
Extremities: Claws on hands and feet, quadrupeds (walk on all fours)

Omnivore
Includes: Dogs, hogs, chickens, bears, etc.
Diet: Meat, vegetables, fruits, roots
Digestive System: Large mouth opening, multi-directional jaw, sharp canine teeth or beaks, moderate to rough tongue, less than or equal to 1 pH with food in stomach, somewhat sacculated small intestine – 4 to 6 times body length, short and smooth colon
Extremities: Hoofs, claws, and paws, quadrupeds (walk on all fours) – except birds.

Herbivore
Includes: Horses, cows, elephants, giraffes, etc.
Diet: Vegetables, herbs, roots, barks
Digestive System: Small mouth opening, multi-directional jaw, broad and flat molars made for grinding – small or no canines, moderately rough tongue, 4 to 5 pH with food in stomach, long and sacculated small intestine – 10 to 12+ times body length, long and sacculated colon
Extremities: hoofs, quadrupeds (walk on all fours)

Frugivore
Includes: Bonobos, Gorillas, Chimpanzees, etc.

Diet: Mainly fruits, leafy greens, vegetables, nuts, seeds
Digestive System: Small mouth opening, multi-directional jaw, usually 32 teeth (including incisors, canines – short and blunted, premolars, and molars), smooth tongue, 4 to 5 pH with food in stomach, long and sacculated small intestine – 10 to 11 times body length, long and sacculated colon
Extremities: Hands with fingers, feet with toes, capable of bipedalism (uses two legs for walking - walks upright)

I had never heard it broken down in this way before, but once I did, it made so much sense. I came to the conclusion that there is only one group of vertebrates that the human species fits into perfectly – Frugivore! A massive light went off in my mind and my world view completely changed.

To be clear - being a frugivore, as shown above, does not mean that we only eat fruit – but that we would generally prefer fruit over other options, when available. Every species on the planet seeks the food that their body is physiologically designed to digest, absorb, utilize, and eliminate the most efficiently – nature always seeks efficiency. For humans, that food is fruit, as it takes very little effort for the body to break it down and utilize its energy.

Fruit is full of simple sugars, vitamins, minerals, antioxidants, polyphenols, hydration, prebiotic fiber, and other phytochemicals that help to power our brain and nervous system. We have color vision to help us spot a ripe apple, mango, or strawberry while out in nature. Our sense of smell is calibrated to generate arousal from the tantalizing fragrances of fruits and berries. Our hands are perfectly formed to pluck fruits from a tree, and our fingers to peel them. And we have a smooth tongue that is designed to enjoy the sweet flavors of fruits (and vegetables).

On the other hand, we are disgusted by the sight and smell of a bloody carcass and deeply disturbed by the sound of an animal in pain. Have you ever lost your appetite after finding a random hair in your meal? These kinds of things would not bother an animal that was meant to eat the flesh of other animals.

To further reinforce this idea, I began making a mental list of all the foods that I could eat with absolute enjoyment, in their most natural form, without cooking, seasoning, marinating, or any other alterations. The thought of biting into the leg of a rabbit or a cow did not seem appetizing at all. Not to mention, the potential risk of being bitten, scratched, or trampled while trying to catch these wild animals did not seem pleasant.

I then changed my focus to foods that would not run away or become aggressive towards me. I imagined sinking my teeth into a ripe peach picked right from the tree and my mouth immediately began to salivate. If you have ever eaten a freshly picked, tree ripened peach or mango, you would immediately appreciate the absolute perfect communion between humans and fruit. These are the foods that we can most easily obtain, and they are perfectly suited to the human anatomy and physiology. This would explain why I have never needed to add salt or sugar to a piece of fruit - it is already perfectly designed for my enjoyment.

With all of that said, it is still important to include a variety of other whole plant foods, especially leafy greens, colorful vegetables, herbs, sea vegetables, and some nuts and seeds. Eating a diet of only fruit, especially from our current agricultural system, is not something that I would recommend doing - due to fruits being harvested unripe, poor farming practices, potentially depleted soils, and other factors.

With all of that, I thought I had been exposed to everything I needed to know about why I should be eating more fruits and vegetables - but I was about to experience my third shift in consciousness that would change the way I looked at animals.

I became aware of a documentary called "Earthlings." It revealed undercover footage of how animals are used and objectified in the production of food, clothing, and entertainment. At this point, I had already begun dramatically shifting my diet to include more plants and less animal products but solely from a health perspective. This opened my eyes to the ethical implications of consuming and using animal products. I remember laying on my bed watching in shock and disbelief as I witnessed the reality of what I had been contributing to through my diet and lifestyle choices.

With my newfound awareness of animal sentience and the inherent suffering associated with animal products - combined with what I was learning about the nutritional requirements of the human body - I was confronted with my own cognitive dissonance surrounding my lifestyle choices and the only logical choice was to adopt a whole food, _vegan_ lifestyle.

I still remember the last bite of meat that I ever had. I was driving home from work and out of habit, I found myself pulling into the drive-up of one of my favorite fast food restaurants. I ordered my usual two cheeseburgers and when I removed the first burger from the bag and took my first bite, I was hit with a sobering dose of cognitive dissonance.

I thought of the individual animal that suffered and died to make the burger I held. I also had a visualization of the chemicals and preservatives from the meat and cheese being incorporated into my body and the inflammatory effects that would ensue. With that one bite still in my mouth, I spit it out, and threw the burgers in the trash - never to consume animal products again.

Since that day, my experiences and research have only reinforced what I now sincerely believe to be the optimal diet (whole food, raw vegan) and lifestyle for human health and the overall well being of animals and the environment. Over the last decade, I have been able to transform and align my body, mind, and spirit to a frequency of health, freedom, and empowerment with a raw vegan diet - and I'm going to show you how you can too!

But Why Raw?

Raw foods contain all of the enzymes, intact fiber, hydration, microbiota, antioxidants, vitamins, and life force that they were endowed with by the Earth. This is the most natural form that we can incorporate these foods into our bodies and once you experience an all (or mostly) raw diet, you will understand the energetic difference between a cooked diet and a raw diet.

When we apply high-heat to a food, it alters the chemical structure to something that the body was not necessarily designed to recognize. Heat takes the life out of the food and necessitates much more energy output from the body to utilize and eliminate these foods.

You might be reading this book to learn how to eat more raw food - but what I think you really want is *the feeling* of health and happiness that can be experienced when we align our actions with a higher vibrational way of living. The truth is, the magic is not *just* in the raw vegan diet but in the synergistic effects of a healthy diet, conscious lifestyle, good relationships, positive mindset, and supporting the body's detoxification processes.

Throughout this program I will teach you to eat a raw vegan diet successfully, but I'm going to let you in on a secret - that's the easy part! Where most people struggle is knowing how to effectively navigate the emotions, social aspects, cravings, and self-sabotage. To create a lasting change in something as deeply ingrained in our subconscious identity as our diet, we must take a holistic and intentional approach - and I will teach you how to do that too!

My goal for this book is <u>not</u> to convince you to do a juice fast or follow my exact daily routine - but to empower you with an easy-to-follow transformational program that is rooted in the five foundational principles of aligning one's body, mind, and spirit, so you can achieve long lasting health and happiness.

The program is set up in a way that puts you in control of personalizing your plan in the best way that you see fit for your unique circumstances. This is not a one-size-fits-all program. Everyone will have their own unique path through the program and will have the autonomy to transition and progress at a speed that is practical and sustainable for them.

So, welcome to the 21-Day Raw Transformation Program - let's have some fun!

The Keys to Transformational Change

Change is an inevitable part of life. We all experience it, but not everyone handles it as well as they'd like to. So, if you struggle with making lasting change to any aspect of your life (like diet) - this program has you covered!

The first thing to consider is if you are open to change in the first place. You're reading this book, so there is a good chance you have reached a point in your life where you feel a change is needed.

The next thing to determine is the type of lens that you choose to perceive the events in your life. There are two basic lenses of perception that a person will use to observe their life through - **extrinsic or intrinsic**.

Someone with an **extrinsic perception** of life believes that whatever happens to them is predominantly due to external factors. If they get fired from their job or fail an exam, they blame the people around them or their circumstances for why these things happened to them. In other words, they see themselves as being at the mercy of their environment.

On the other hand, someone perceiving life from an **intrinsic lens** is someone who believes that *they* themselves are ultimately responsible for whatever happens in their life. They are the captain of their ship and embrace the idea that they can create any outcome they desire - when they take the necessary action.

The person looking through an intrinsic lens can recognize that they have the power to create deep, meaningful change - regardless of their current circumstances. The kind of change that illuminates their body, mind, and spirit. Change that is so transformative that they practically have to reintroduce themselves to their friends and family.

So, which lens have you been looking through? If you feel that now is the time to make transformational change in your life - then I invite you to evaluate your perception of life and the role you play in achieving your goals.

When you fully embrace the intrinsic mindset that your actions are the primary factor in determining how much your life will change - for better or worse - then you have liberated yourself from victimhood and stepped into a place of power and creation.

From that point, it is just a matter of recognizing which aspects of your life that need to change for you to experience the highest level of positive transformation - and taking action to learn and implement those changes.

The *21-Day Raw Transformation Program* is designed to help you do just that. You will be guided through five core pillars of transformational change:

Conscious Shift
Dietary Design
Lifestyle Basics
Detoxification Optimization
Support Systems

This program is not just about changing your diet or exercise habits. You must change the way you define food, establish strategic boundaries to guide your choices, design a robust support system, and so much more.

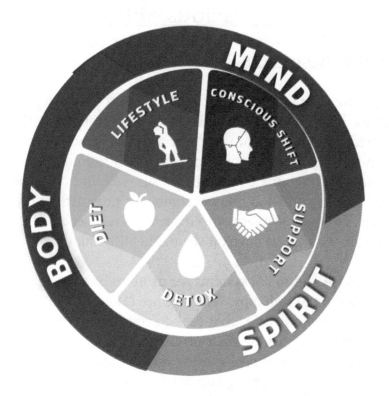

By enhancing these core pillars in your life, you will more closely align your body, mind, and spirit - bringing you the clarity that is needed to make life-long transformational change.

Conscious Shift

Gaining Awareness

Before we start talking about food, we must first recognize that we have been programmed since birth to think and act in certain ways. Unfortunately, for many of us, we have received programming that leads us to self-sabotage. Whether through toxic food, drugs, sex, self-limiting beliefs, emotional suppression, blame, shame, or procrastination - the environment of Westernized societies has become increasingly unfit to develop strong, healthy minds.

Our culture and social systems set us up to be sick, dependent, and unhappy. What we are taught is heavily influenced by industries that seek to condition us to unconsciously consume their products and ideas. Very little importance is placed on fostering health or empowering individuals to develop a genuine relationship with who they are. Instead of helping people develop and express their unique creativity, the system is designed to homogenize the population and constantly distract individuals from ever truly connecting with their authentic self.

As Aristotle said, **"Give me a child until he is seven and I will show you the man."** The foundation of what we believe as adults was programmed into us as children. According to Dr. Bruce Lipton, until around the age of seven, the brain is functioning largely in a theta state, which is associated with imagination and hypnosis. Being in a theta state is like having the record button pushed on the subconscious mind. And because our thoughts literally create our reality, how our life unfolds will largely depend upon the belief systems and thought programs that we were given within the first decade of our life - unless we become conscious of our subconscious programming and work to rewrite the programs.

Dr. Lipton and other researchers have found that out of the many thousands of thoughts that run through a person's mind each day, only about 5% of them are done so in the conscious (creative) mind. The conscious mind is where your desires and aspirations are held. Your desire to adopt a raw vegan diet and lifestyle is in your conscious mind.

The other 95% of our thoughts are generated from the unconscious (habitual) mind. This is where our habitual thoughts, beliefs, and actions are kept, which will take over when the conscious mind is not actively engaged. These habitual subconscious programs are mostly what we picked up as children in the theta brain state and as adults they act as an autopilot program that helps us to function effortlessly throughout the day without actively thinking about every detail of what we do.

Furthermore, even the thoughts that we create from the conscious mind are filtered through our subconscious programming and if the new thoughts are not compatible with the established programs, then those thoughts can be instantaneously modified to fit within the old subconscious framework - similar to an autocorrect program on your computer.

I'll give you an example: At the gym where I work out, they have an Announcements Board where there is a big, bright sign announcing "Pizza Party Fridays" for all members - it's a very popular event. In a place where people go to lose weight and get healthy, they celebrate their efforts by consuming something that will keep them from losing weight and getting healthy. This perfectly shows the collective subconscious programming that runs our society, where the person's conscious mind says, "I want to get healthy," but their subconscious (habitual) mind says, "I love junk food" or "Everything in moderation" and sabotages their efforts.

The reason that I never even considered eating the pizza is because I updated my subconscious definition of what food is - and conventional pizza does not fit that description in my program's dictionary anymore. However, most of the other members were still operating from a program that recognized things like pizza and bagels as food for the human body - and so it was well within their parameters to eat pizza as a reward for exercising.

So, when someone says to me, "Wow, that's great that you can eat so healthy, but I don't have the willpower to do that," what they are actually saying is, "I wish I could eat healthily, but my subconscious programming keeps me from doing so." If you have been trying and trying to change your diet or lifestyle and you keep struggling to make lasting changes, then you know that your subconscious programs are not in alignment with your conscious desires to change.

If you want to succeed at changing your diet and lifestyle for the long term, you must become aware of the subconscious programs that are controlling 95% of your thoughts, beliefs, and actions. Once you have this awareness, you can then work on evaluating and modifying those programs to more closely align with the intentions in your conscious mind. When this is done, you will find that you experience much greater success with making these diet and lifestyle modifications.

Changing The Environment

Another important step that we must take to shift our state of consciousness and overcome old programming is to <u>change the internal and external environments</u> that we expose ourselves to on a daily basis. We have the external environment that we are exposed to from the outside world, and we also have the internal environment that we create with our thoughts and perceptions. Most of society is operating within a fear-based paradigm that permeates their internal and external environments and keeps them perpetually stressed, hyper-reactive, self-critical, and short-sighted.

When we operate in a fear-based paradigm we tend to view ourselves with a victim mentality. You have probably known a family where every one is overweight with similar health issues and they tell you that these things run in their family and there is nothing that they can do about it - this is an example of subconscious victim-based programming. In reality, everyone in this family has been exposed to the same environments (food, lifestyle, beliefs, thought patterns) and so they display the same or similar results in their lives. If they became aware that they are just running a subconscious program and that they actually have a great deal of control over how their life unfolds, then they could work to rewrite their programming and create a different reality for themselves.

70% of the average person's subconscious thoughts are negative, repetitive, and self-limiting. This is important to recognize because negative thinking impacts a person's reality just as much as positive thinking does - and because 95% of our overall thoughts and actions come from the subconscious mind, rewiring any fear-based or victim-based thought programs that we were given as children (or adults) should be a top priority.

So, why is it so difficult for people to see that their subconscious programming is sabotaging their happiness and success? Fear activates the sympathetic nervous system (fight or flight) and suppresses a person's ability to rationally evaluate the situation that they are in. A fearful mind is constantly in a state of survival which increases stress hormones and drastically reduces a person's overall awareness and forethought. And unfortunately, our society appears designed to bombard us with messages of fear from every angle (terrorism, disease, bills, climate change, the economy, etc.).

It is much easier to manipulate and control a person who is in a fearful state and industry marketers and news organizations take full advantage of this. This is why the vast majority of news reports are negative and you see the same television commercials playing repeatedly. They know that repetition - especially in a stressed and fearful mind - can more easily train a person's subconscious mind to accept the messages being presented on the screen. Additionally, prolonged fear wears down and disempowers a person to believe that the solution to their problems can only be found outside of themself - which means someone or something else holds the power to their happiness or freedom.

This is why we must be especially mindful of the external messaging that we allow into our eyes and ears - whether it comes from friends, colleagues, family, the news, music, magazines, books, movies, gurus, or social media - it all has an impact on our subconscious programming. You might be reading this book to help you change the foods you choose to put into your mouth, but first, you must ensure that your subconscious programming is compatible with your conscious desire to change. If not, your habitual subconscious mind will work against you when your conscious mind is distracted by other things, and it will be far more difficult to make lasting change in anything that you do.

So, take an inventory of what you are feeding your mind through your eyes and ears and be intentional about upgrading the environments that you place yourself in. When we do this, we can more easily eliminate the fear and move into a love-based state of consciousness, which expands our scope of awareness and it becomes much easier to see ourselves as a creator of our circumstances rather than a victim of them. In a love-based state of awareness, we are more capable of taping into our intuition. We gain a higher level of compassion and empathy for ourselves and others which deepens our connection with all life and illuminates that everything around us is a mere extension of the self - like different fingers on the same hand.

The more we take steps to construct a supportive external environment, the easier it will be to elevate the quality of our internal dialogue - which will lead us to feel more empowered and allow us to make better choices with our diet and anything else that we desire. As they say, we are a product of the five people that we hang around the most - so choose wisely who you allow into your inner circle and the environments that you place yourself in. We will touch more on this later in the book when we discuss the importance of building healthy support systems.

Incredible blessings and synchronicities can be experienced when we reach an internal state of love-consciousness in combination with a supportive external environment. This creates a powerful feedback loop where the internal and external environments nourish and strengthen each other. In this state you are better able to handle and process any difficulties that may arise in your life. You will begin finding silver linings and opportunities in the challenges that used to upset and dishearten you. And during times of emotional hardship, a healthy inner circle will be there to pick you up and support you when you need it. It all works together beautifully.

So the take away message is this: A shift in consciousness is a prerequisite to creating any lasting change in our lives. We must gain an awareness of the subconscious programming that we received as children and update those programs if necessary. Our internal and external environments and our perception of reality will either work for us or against us in making the changes that we desire in our conscious mind. Information must transfer from the conscious mind to the subconscious mind in order for our desires to manifest in our life.

For example, as we see with New Year's resolutions, it is possible to stick to a new diet or exercise routine for while - but if this new information or action has not been installed in the person's subconscious programming, it will not last long term. This is why the gyms are half empty after March. So, if you want to be successful with the raw vegan diet and lifestyle, then you have to also expand your consciousness and your perception of reality to allow for this information to be compatible with your subconscious programming.

Putting It Into Practice:

1. Gain Awareness

Before you can change something, you must first become aware of it. Be mindful of any habitual thought patterns or actions that you feel interfere with your success of changing your diet and lifestyle.

Utilize meditation and introspection to gain awareness of these things. Write them down and take note of the emotions that are connected to them to help you understand the tiggers and potential solutions for change.

For example, if you always find that you eat a bowl of ice cream at night after you've had a stressful day, write it down. Once you have this awareness of these habits, you can work on finding solutions to replace them with something more beneficial.

In the above example, identifying the source of stress would be a good place to start. From there you can evaluate what options you have to reduce or eliminate that source of stress. And of course replace the conventional ice cream with banana nice cream so you are nourishing the body rather than obstructing it.

2.   Re-evaluate your belief systems

With awareness and introspection of our conscious and subconscious belief systems, we can begin to evaluate what we currently believe about the raw vegan diet and lifestyle and determine which beliefs align with truth, where we may need more research, and what information can be discarded or replaced.

For example: If you still believe that plants are inherently deficient in essential nutrients or that it is too difficult to eat a raw diet because of x, y, and z - then you must take a deeper look into why you hold these beliefs and if they hold up under scrutiny. Is it possible that you are just repeating a subconscious thought program that you picked up from someone else who holds a limiting belief? Is there perhaps an alternate conclusion that could be made if you had more information?

You must have the humility to consider that your current belief systems could be inaccurate. Research all sides of the issue and be open to changing your stance based on new evidence and insights.

Most of all, be truly honest with yourself and always stay curious.

3. Recalibrate The Subconscious Mind

The subconscious mind is also known as the habitual mind. It runs our habits through the programs that we download from our environment. We receive the foundation of our subconscious programming throughout the first seven years of life when the brain is operating predominantly in a theta wave state. During this time, we unconsciously download these programs from our parents, teachers, coaches, friends, neighbors, television, and everything else that we were exposed to as young children.

Once we gain awareness of the programs that we have been given, there are several techniques that Dr. Bruce Lipton recommends for rewriting our reprogramming. Here are two ways that he promotes anyone can easily start with:

Self-hypnosis: After the age of 7, the brain enters the theta wave state much less often. However, we do reach theta at least twice each day - as we are falling asleep and as we are waking up from sleep. In the moments before falling asleep your brain goes into a theta state and is much more suggestible to hypnosis and subconscious programming. Each night as you are falling asleep (and in the first hour after waking), you can listen to a recording of affirmations or other information that you want to download into your subconscious programming.

You can use your phone, a tape player, or voice recording device to play these messages to your subconscious mind while you are falling asleep and going through the theta state each night.

Repetition: After the age of seven, one of the best ways to program the subconscious mind is through practice and repetition. In the same way that you learn to play an instrument or drive a car as an adult - practicing over and over until it becomes a natural habit - you can train your subconscious through repeated exposure to a desired message or action that you want to install into your subconscious habits.

A great place to begin on your raw vegan journey is committing to have a fruit smoothie as your first meal of the day for at least 21 days and soon it will be a natural routine that you do automatically. Later in this book, I will give you additional guidance on some easy plans that you can follow each day and turn healthy eating into a repeatable habit.

4. Master Your Attention

While you're in the process of rewriting your mental programming - think of your conscious mind as a plot of fertile soil, and your thoughts as the seeds that you plant in the soil. The quality of the seeds (thoughts) that you plant in your mind will determine the quality of your experiences. However, just planting the seed does not guarantee that it will grow. Your attention is the greatest factor in determining which of these seeds will sprout.

Attention is a powerful energy that waters the seeds in your conscious mind. Without your attention, the thoughts in your conscious mind will not grow long enough roots to reach the subconscious mind and, therefore will have limited power to manifest into your reality.

Be aware that other entities, such as corporations, desperately try to capture your attention and influence your behavior. If you learn to control your attention, you reclaim an enormous amount of power to take control of your life.

Keep in mind that the water, seeds, and soil alone are not enough to produce a healthy plant – you also need the right amount of sunshine. Your spoken word is like the powerful sun, shining a full spectrum of energy and life force for your seedlings to absorb. The higher the quality of your spoken word - towards yourself and everyone else - the healthier and stronger your seedlings will become.

We currently have a rising epidemic of toxic, low quality language that is feeding the weeds in people's minds. Fueled largely by television, music, and other media sources, the way people have learned to speak to themselves and others has regressed into a self-limiting, culturally dividing exercise. Be mindful of how you are using language and determine whether you are nurturing your seeds or your weeds.

After all of that – you may have great soil, quality seeds, just the right amount of water and sunshine, but if you are planting in the wrong climate, your seeds will STILL not produce the desired results. For example, planting a perfect mango seed in the rich, healthy soil of an organic Minnesota farm with plenty of water and sunshine will not produce a healthy, fruitful mango tree.

The climate in which you plant your "mental seeds" is represented by the action that you take to grow them. You might have a healthy mindset, positive thoughts, focused attention, and use high quality language, but if you fail to take the necessary action required to bring your conscious mind's thoughts and desires into fruition, you might as well be planting the perfect mango seed in Minnesota.

To summarize – it is not enough to just think positive thoughts or repeat affirmations to yourself. To greatly increase the odds of achieving any goal, it is essential to bring these five principles together:

Growth-oriented mindset (healthy soil) – Believe that you can achieve anything you put your mind to.
Healthy thoughts (seeds) – Think positive, empowering thoughts about yourself, your goals, and others.
Focused attention (water) – Remove the distractions and stay focused on your goals.
High-quality language (sunshine) – Speak kindly to yourself and others. Words are powerful – use them wisely.
Action/follow-through (climate) – Nobody is going to do the work for you. Put in the work and make your dreams happen.

Neglecting just one of these principles can cause dreams and aspirations to go unrealized. How many people do you know that have amazing ideas but are never focused enough to follow through with them? What about the people that always speak poorly of themselves or others – do you see them achieving many of their goals?

This world can be a tough place to live, which is why you need to be your biggest supporter! If you do not support yourself, why would anyone else? Your environment responds to the energy you send out with your words, thoughts, and emotions. Live with conviction and integrity, and your experience in life will be so much more rewarding.

You are truly capable of creating unlimited possibilities, and you have everything you need within you to achieve whatever you desire. The more you believe this, the easier things will fall into place for you. This book is your blueprint to getting your diet, lifestyle, and state of mind where you need them, so you have the energy and focus to create your most authentic life possible!

5. Think in Terms of Frequency

Finally, start to see things in terms of frequency. Everything holds a frequency - you, me, our cells, animals, plants, water, the Earth, thoughts, emotions, intentions, words, actions, etc.

Have you ever met someone that makes you feel good or uplifted just by being around them? Maybe you've felt the energy be sucked out of a room once someone walked in. You are picking up on their frequency!

We tend to synchronize our own frequency with those of the things we consume (food, media, ideas, etc.) - as well as what is in our environment (people, plants, nature, etc.) So, it is very important to be mindful of what we expose ourselves to if we want to achieve a higher frequency.

Truth, love, joy, laughter, optimism, acts of kindness, good intentions, fruits, vegetables, and clean water are all examples of things that carry a high frequency.

Fear, anger, shame, jealousy, hate, gossip, deceit, lying, harming ourselves or others, suffering, unethical behavior, processed junk foods, synthetic chemicals, pollution, and stealing are examples of things with low frequency.

Start surrounding yourself with more high frequencies and be intentional about limiting or eliminating the low frequencies you currently have in your life.

Dietary Design

There is no shortage of opinions regarding the best way to structure a raw vegan diet. Some say the diet should be high in fat, some advocate low fat, some groups eat mostly sprouts and greens, while others eat mostly fruit. There are also disagreements about whether cooked foods have a role to play in someone's diet. Some will say that all cooked foods are poison and others believe that some cooked foods can be a healthy addition to a mostly raw diet. So, how do we determine which style is right for us?

I don't believe that it is appropriate nor practical to use a broad brush to paint the exact same raw food diet for everyone. There are many factors (geographical, financial, etc.) that play a part in determining the dietary approach that will best meet an individual's various needs while also being a sustainable way of life. Of course, there are principles in this program that work great for most people - but everyone's path will be slightly different - so this is an opportunity for you to create a unique plan that works for YOU.

I designed the 21-Day Raw Transformation Program based on my personal experience over the last ten years of experimenting with the various styles of raw vegan dietary approaches and forming a style that I could easily maintain. I have taken that practice and experience and built a system around it that I believe anyone can be successful with. The key is to keep things simple enough that it is easy to follow, diverse enough to keep it enjoyable, and flexible enough to fit into anyone's life.

General Dietary Guidelines

The 21-Day Raw Transformation Program offers two paths that you can choose to take when designing your raw vegan diet:

1. **All Raw**: For those who desire to eat only raw foods.

2. **High Raw:** For those who desire to eat primarily raw foods (roughly 80% of daily calories or more), with the addition of small amounts of cooked, whole plant foods.

Regardless of which path you choose, the foundation of the program is built upon an abundance of fruits throughout the first half of the day for hydration and energy and a large 5-Star Salad in the afternoon for balance and stability.

It is essential that you stick to these two foundational aspects of the plan. Especially for those that choose the "High Raw" path - be intentional about getting in the full amount of raw food that is laid out in the guidelines when any cooked food is included.

Low Fat (10-20% of overall calories): When you eat a diet of primarily raw fruits and vegetables, you will naturally consume a relatively low amount of fat - which I believe is critical to long-term success. By following the suggested meal plan, you should fall somewhere between 10-20% of overall calories coming from fat. This will help support optimal insulin sensitivity in your body and allow for the proper regulation of blood glucose when consuming a higher level of carbohydrates from fruits and vegetables.

Omega Conscious: I refer to the balance of omega-6 to omega-3 fats in someone's diet as their omega fatty acid ratio (OFAR), which ideally we want in the range of 1:1 to 4:1. Most people are eating far too many omega-6 fats (vegetable oils, processed foods, etc.) in comparison to their omega-3 fat (flax, chia, hemp, walnuts, leafy greens) intake - often giving them an OFAR score of 15:1 or higher!

The proper balance of omega-6 to omega-3 is essential for regulating inflammation in the body, promoting the conversion and generation of long-chain fats like EPA and DHA, and maintaining healthy immune and nervous system function. Because omega-6 and omega-3 fats compete for the same enzymes that convert them into their elongated forms (AA, EPA, DHA), I encourage the addition of 1 - 2 tsps of ground flax or chia seeds in your breakfast smoothie each day. This gets a substantial amount of omega-3 fats into the system to hopefully be converted to EPA and DHA before any concentrated sources of omega-6 fats are consumed.

Fats After Four: All overt fats (avocado, nuts, seeds, etc.) - with the exception of 1 - 2 tsp of flax or chia seeds in your breakfast smoothie - should be consumed with the dinner salad in the afternoon. Fats take the longest of all the macronutrients to digest, so to optimize your digestion throughout the day, it can be beneficial to consume fats after 4:00 pm, when you have dinner.

Eating a significant amount of fat early in the day can lead to gas, bloating, and indigestion later in the day when faster digesting foods are eaten.

Fruits First, Salad Second: Another general guideline to support proper digestion is to eat fruits in the first part of the day (or meal) and the more dense foods, like salads and vegetables in the second part of the day. This keeps the fastest digesting foods out in front of the slower digesting foods to have a clean, steady flow of digestion.

Eat It Ripe Or Go On Strike: It is absolutely critical to have access to - and know how to select quality, ripe fruits. If you attempt to eat a raw vegan diet with unripe, low-quality fruits, you will struggle to find enjoyment in it.

Talk to your produce people or if you're fortunate enough to know the farmers - have them show you how to pick out the best produce. Each fruit is different, but in general, fruits should be brightly colored, fragrant, and slightly soft but not too soft.

Also, take advantage of Asian Markets if you have one in your community - they usually have a good variety of different fruits that you won't find in your average grocery store.

If you do not have access to a good variety of quality fruits, I would recommend utilizing more frozen fruits or eating more vegetables and greens. Many people in this type of situation will do better on the "High Raw" path until their circumstances change.

Start The Day With Water: We lose a significant amount of water throughout the night as we sleep. A great way to replace this lost hydration is by starting the day with 32oz of clean water. This helps to rehydrate the body and flush the system of toxins that the body had designated for elimination over the night. Feel free to add fresh lemon to your water if desired. Distilled or reverse osmosis water is recommended.

Snacking: In the meal plan menu there are several snack recipes that you can make but I encourage you to utilize fresh fruit (apples, oranges, etc.) as your main snack of choice. Snacks such as fruit can be enjoyed throughout the day as much as needed - no limitations - but it is recommended to avoid eating snacks after dinner to prevent indigestion.

Organic When Possible: The more we can avoid synthetic chemicals (i.e. pesticides), the better off we will be. Many synthetic pesticides are neurotoxic, meaning they can damage the brain and nervous system - as well as our gut health. They can also have endocrine-disrupting effects, which cause problems with the organs and glands that regulate our hormones. So, not only is this better for our overall health, but it also makes the food we eat so much more flavorful and nutritious!

If eating 100% organic is not a practical option for you at this point, I recommend utilizing the Environmental Working Group's *Dirty Dozen* and *Clean Fifteen* lists to help you make the best choices when deciding which foods to buy organic.

I strongly encourage avoiding all genetically modified (GMO) foods, such as non-organic corn, soy, canola oil, cottonseed oil, white sugar (sugar beets), Hawaii-grown papayas, pink flesh pineapples, summer squash, and others. The safest way to avoid GMO ingredients is to buy organic as much as you can and by avoiding all processed foods.

If Cooked Food Is Consumed, It Must Be Eaten With A Large Raw Salad:

If you are choosing the "High Raw" path on this program, then I ask that you commit to only eating cooked food during dinner and always with or after a big leafy green salad. This provides you with additional hydration and bioactive enzymes that will help you better digest the cooked food.

Setting Your Boundaries

To help you build a sustainable framework for your raw vegan diet, The 21-Day Raw Transformation Program utilizes a traffic light system to give you a clear understanding of which foods should generally be used to make up the core or foundation of your diet, which foods should be used in a supportive manner, and which foods should be avoided completely. The Traffic Light System will help you define your dietary boundaries in a way that is specific, yet flexible so

TRAFFIC LIGHT SYSTEM

GREEN LIGHT
CORE FOODS

Fruits and berries (all edible kinds)	Jicama
Green leafy vegetables	Kohlrabi
Non-starchy vegetables	Leeks
Asparagus	Mushrooms
Beets	Okra
Brussel sprouts	Onions
Broccoli	Peppers
Carrots	Pea pods
Cauliflower	Radishes
Celery	Sprouts/microgreens
Cucumber	Tomato
Herbal teas	Water chestnuts
Herbs and spices	Clean Water

YELLOW LIGHT
SUPPORT FOODS

Should be eaten raw:
- Avocado
- Coconut
- Dehydrated & Dried Foods
- Olives (not packed in oil)
- Nuts
- Seeds
- Sea vegetables
  - Wakame, Dulse, Nori, Kelp
- Condiments
  - Carob, Cacao, Maple Syrup, Nutritional Yeast, Sea Salt, Raw Plant Milks, Seed Cheeses

Typically eaten cooked:
- Beans & Lentils
- Steamed Vegetables & Squash
- Corn (can also be eaten raw)
- Potatoes of all types
- Pseudo Grains
  - Amaranth, Buckwheat, Quinoa, etc.
- Rice (Brown, White, Wild, etc.)
- Tofu, Tempeh, & Other Soy Products
- Condiments & Specialty Items
  - Organic Coffee, Sprouted Breads

RED LIGHT
AVOIDANCE FOODS

Artificial sweeteners (all kinds)	Highly processed meat alternatives
Breads	Meat (all types)
Dairy products (all kinds)	Oils (any kind)
Eggs	Pastries
Fish and seafood	Processed meats
Fried foods	Refined sugars
High fructose corn syrup	Genetic & Modified Organisms (GMOs)

you do not feel restricted.

Let's take a closer look at the three categories:

Green Light Foods (core foods)

The Green Light category contains foods that can be enjoyed in abundance and should make up the majority of your diet. These foods are raw, nutrient-dense, fiber-rich, hydrating, and generally easy to digest and eliminate. Green light foods should be eaten in their whole food form – meaning, they should always be unprocessed or at most, minimally processed. They typically do not come in a package or a box (unless you buy by the case!) and never require an ingredients list. These are your core foods.

Yellow Light Foods (support foods)

The Yellow Light category is comprised of foods that are still generally healthy whole plant foods, but should be consumed in smaller amounts, or as needed, to play a supporting role in your diet. The amount of support foods in your diet will depend on your personal goals as well as what is practical, given your individual circumstances.

As indicated in the list above, Yellow Light foods are divided into "raw" and "consciously cooked" options. Nuts, seeds, and fatty fruits should always be eaten raw to preserve the integrity of the delicate fatty acids. When fatty acids are heated, they oxidize and become rancid, leading to oxidative stress and inflammation in the body.

For those that choose to take the "High Raw" path and include small amounts of consciously cooked whole foods with their dinner salad - I want to emphasize the term **"conscious cooking."** This refers to using cooking methods that result in the least amount of damaging effects to the food - such as steaming, boiling, and pressure cooking.

Cooking with dry heat, such as baking, grilling, or frying, creates higher levels of harmful byproducts like advanced glycation end products (AGEs), polycyclic aromatic hydrocarbons (PAHs), and acrylamide that can damage DNA and promote disease - these cooking methods should be avoided as much as possible.

When adding consciously cooked ingredients to a dinner salad, there are a few guidelines to follow:

1. **Consciously cooked food should always be eaten with a large, raw salad.**
   This ensures you consume additional hydration and enzymes to promote proper digestion and elimination.

2. **Consciously cooked foods should always be eaten in their whole food form - or at most, minimally processed.**
   Processed foods contain addictive, hyper-stimulating additives (salt, sugar, oil, flavorings) that desensitize our taste buds to the flavors of natural fruits and vegetables. This leads people to crave these artificial stimulations and become less interested in healthy foods.

   Stick to whole foods that you prepare at home where you control what is added to the dish. If needed - use herbs and spices rather than salt to bring out more flavor in your meals.

3. **Consciously cooked food should never displace fresh, raw, Green Light foods from your diet.**
   Cooked foods should always be used in a supporting role, not as a replacement. Be intentional about consistently consuming enough fresh, raw fruits and vegetables to fulfill as much of your needs as possible and from there fill in the gaps with your consciously cooked whole foods.

You should always be getting in your smoothie for breakfast, fruits throughout the middle part of the day, and your 5-Star Salad for dinner. After that - on the "High Raw" plan - you can enjoy as much consciously cooked whole foods as is needed to fully satisfy your needs.

Red Light Foods (avoidance foods)

Some things should just not be considered food – red light "foods" are just that. These items are either high in saturated and trans fat, void of fiber, highly contaminated with toxins, highly processed, or highly inflammatory, which all promote disease in the body. Do your best to completely avoid the items on this list as much as you can.

Using The Traffic Light System

Have you ever been driving somewhere in a hurry, and you keep getting stopped, one red light after another? Talk about frustrating! On the other hand, have you ever experienced the thrill of seeing every traffic light you approach turn green, allowing you to seamlessly navigate toward your destination? In this case, your desired health is the destination you are "driving" towards, and you have the power to influence the flow of traffic based on the foods you choose to eat.

Sticking with the car analogy – to get the best gas mileage out of your car, you need to drive in a controlled manner and at a consistent speed. If you constantly speed up and slow down erratically, you are going to burn through your gas very quickly and end up stranded on the side of the road and probably blaming the car for failing you when it was just how you were driving it!

Using that same line of thinking, you will maximize the benefit and satisfaction you receive from your diet by staying relatively consistent and under control, rather than flip-flopping back and forth between different dietary programs or styles of eating. I have noticed that people who frequently make dramatic changes to their dietary approach have a hard time achieving the health they desire, and they typically implement "cheat days" or "cheat meals" just so that they can stick to their current program.

By setting strategic boundaries with your yellow light foods and sticking to general guidelines of the plan, you will significantly reduce the risk or desire for "cheat days" because your dietary approach no longer feels rigid or restrictive. You now have ample options that will keep you within the framework of your plan without sacrificing your health or the progress you have made.

When someone makes a habit of permitting "cheat days" where they periodically indulge on red light foods that are counterproductive to their goals, this can lead to undesirable microbiome alterations, weight gain, bingeing, and increased cravings. Cheat days only cheat yourself, and even if nobody else sees you do it – as Dr. Michael Klaper says – "your body is never not looking!" **The goal is to create a way of eating (and thinking) that you love so much that there is no desire to fill your divine body with harmful substances in the first place – I believe you will find this with the 21-Day Raw Transformation Program.**

Keeping A Healthy Mindset Around Food

I believe a great advantage to using the Traffic Light System is that it helps a person establish positive emotional boundaries around food. While I am a staunch advocate of as many raw fruits and vegetables in a person's diet as possible, I do not believe that it creates a healthy relationship with food to perceive eating a steamed potato as an unhealthy failure.

But I get it – one hundred percent raw is sexy, and maintaining an all raw diet is a great accomplishment in the challenging societal systems that we live in. And especially for someone dealing with a high priority health condition, one hundred percent raw may be the most appropriate approach and mindset to have. However, for the average person, who is just trying to learn how to eat more healthfully, some steamed vegetables with their salad might be precisely what they need to prevent them from making an ACTUAL unhealthy food choice.

With that said - please, do not use that as an excuse to settle for anything less than your best effort. If you are in a position to maintain an all raw diet and that is your goal, then stick with it - but use this as a reminder to stay practical and compassionate with yourself on this journey. Most of us are not living in an ideal environment, social network, or culture that makes healthful living easy - and the fact that you are here right now, reading this book shows a level of commitment to yourself and your happiness that deserves recognition.

The key to your success is not always being perfect but creating a support system for yourself that makes failure virtually impossible – that is what I hope tools like the Raw Intuition Traffic Light System will do for you.

The 5-Yes Test

The 5-Yes Test is a tool that is designed to help you determine which foods (and meals) should make up the bulk of the green light and yellow light foods in your program. Green Light foods should get a "yes" to all five questions. Yellow Light foods may get 3-4 "yes" answers. Any food or meal that receives 2 "yes" answers or less should be placed in the Red Light category.

5 YES TEST

1 IS IT HEALTH-PROMOTING?

2 DOES IT TASTE GOOD?

3 DOES IT MAKE ME FEEL GOOD?

4 IS IT AFFORDABLE?

5 DOES IT ELIMINATE WELL?

Not everyone will have the same answers to these questions - because again, everyone is living under different circumstances and we all have access to slightly different foods for a variety of reasons. So, you can use the 5-Yes Test to help you establish personalized boundaries to place in your traffic light system:

1. **Is it health-promoting?**
   Does this food support my long-term health? Is it a natural food? Does it provide the vitamins, minerals, antioxidants, fiber, and other constituents that support the optimal functioning of my body and mind?

2. **Does it taste good?**
   Many people that are trying to eat healthy according to the latest fads are led to believe that they need to consume all sorts of unpalatable concoctions in order to achieve their goals. I believe that we should listen to our

intuition and eat whole foods that naturally taste good to our tongue in order to fuel the body to a healthy state.

One caveat though - many people have perverted their taste buds to such a degree that natural whole foods do not always taste very good. So, in that instance, there may be a grace period where some fruits and vegetables do not provide the same level of satisfaction as the artificially hyper-stimulating foods do. Over time **this will change** and the taste buds will adapt and eventually crave the natural flavors of fresh fruits and vegetables.

3. **Does it make me feel good?**
    A great way to tell if a food or meal should be a part of your regular diet is paying attention to how it makes you feel - both immediately after and over the next few days. Something might taste good, but if you feel tired, irritable, or have other negative symptoms, then it might be a Red Light food for you.

    For example, a high-fat, raw gourmet meal often tastes delicious and satisfying in the moment, however shortly after and even the next day, I feel lethargic, dehydrated, and low energy. So these types of meals would fall into the Yellow Light category for me.

4. **Is it affordable?**
    A food that meets all of the other requirements to be a green light food, but puts a strain on your financial budget - then it should fall into your Yellow Light category. This would be a food that can be enjoyed on occasion but would not be a practical food to buy on a regular basis. For me this would be durian or jackfruit - I absolutely love them, but they are very expensive where I live, so I just enjoy them on special occasions.

Even fresh mango and papaya are quite expensive where I live, so I have to either buy them frozen (this is much more affordable) or I just enjoy them when they are in season or on sale.

5. **Does it eliminate well?**
   One of the most important factors that many people neglect to consider, is how the foods they eat affect their bowel movements. Some foods result in easy, clean bowel movements that require very little clean up (wiping) afterwards. These are generally high water content fruits, vegetables, and tender leafy greens. However, some of the more fatty foods, cooked, and dehydrated foods can slow down a person's elimination and cause bowel movements to leave more residue (to be wiped up) and a more foul smell on their way out.

   Each person will have their own experience with certain foods, so just pay attention to your body's signals and always be mindful of any changes that occur with your elimination. If a certain food causes constipation or other elimination problems, you should consider putting it in the Red Light category - and if desired - as your digestion improves over time, perhaps you can test it again in the future to see if your body handles it better in a healthier state. If it does, you could move that food into the Yellow Light category to enjoy as a support food.

Daily Meal Design

At this point, you should have a pretty good idea of which foods you are going to be eating. The next question is how should you design your meals throughout the day? Once again there is going to be some variation between each individual's exact design that works best for them. However,

there is one simple outline that I want you to focus on and
we will talk about how you can build upon it as much or as
little as you need to throughout the program.

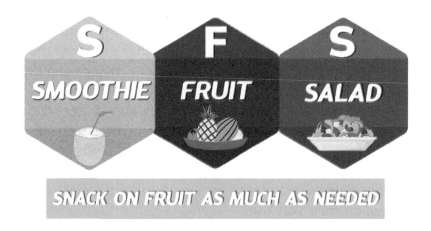

SFS (Smoothie / Fruit / Salad)

The first daily meal design option is SFS - smoothie, fruit,
salad. You might also remember this as "Super freakin'
simple!" This is the general outline that I personally follow
and that has worked amazingly well for me over many years.

Breakfast

Breakfast should always be hydrating and antioxidant-rich.
This supports the brain and nervous system and keeps your
mind clear and sharp throughout the day. It also primes the
body's eliminative pathways to effectively remove waste from
the body and promotes a clean internal environment.

To make things as simplistic as possible, I recommend
starting your day with either smoothies, smoothie bowls, or
whole fresh fruit. Any of these options are a perfect way to

start your day energized and laser-focused on accomplishing your goals.

Make sure to put enough fruit into your smoothies to give you a sufficient amount of calories and keep you satisfied for at least a few hours. My breakfast smoothie usually looks something like this:

7-10 bananas
1-2 cups of a frozen fruit or berry (mango, blueberries, strawberries, cherries, or raspberries)
1-2 tsp of flax or chia seeds (boost of omega-3s)
1-2 cups of a leafy green (kale, spinach, arugula, etc.)
*Sometimes I will add a few sprigs of an herb like basil or cilantro
1-2 cups of distilled water (or to desired consistency)

I usually choose a smoothie for my first meal because it is a fast and simple way to get in an adequate supply of calories, hydration, and nutrition to start my day. This usually satisfies me for 2 - 4 hours before I get hungry again. If you prefer, you can just eat fruit whole (without blending into a smoothie) but for convenience I do recommend smoothies.

Lunch

For lunch, there are a few ways you can go with it. Whichever option you choose, it should always be based around fruit. This can be in the form of a smoothie, smoothie bowl, fruit salad, mono-fruit meal, or a salad with a fat-free, fruit-based dressing. You will find various recipes to choose from in the Meal Plan Menu.

Having a fruit-based lunch will provide you with another supply of calories, nutrition, and hydration to keep you feeling energized and clear-headed throughout the afternoon. No more early afternoon crashes and dozing off at the office after a greasy meal.

I like to keep my lunch meal as simple as possible. Depending on the season, my lunch might look something like this:

5-6 oranges
3-4 Medjool dates
Sometimes, I may also have about a cup of home-grown sprouts (mung bean, alfalfa, lentil, pea, etc.) with some red pepper flakes or other seasonings to finish my lunch meal.

Meals do not have to be complicated. I have come to love simplistic meals during the day. With fruit, you can just peel and eat - it's great.

Dinner

The afternoon or evening meal is where people seem to struggle the most with cravings for old favorites or when they are around friends or family members that are eating a standard diet. That is to be expected, which is why we already covered the importance of changing your consciousness and perspective around food and committing to your health goals.

The great news is that you will be eating a delicious, satisfying 5-Star Salad and homemade dressing **that will make you forget all about those old cravings**! That may seem hard to believe right now, but if you devote the next 21 days to this plan and follow the guidelines, you might be surprised by how much you truly enjoy having a big salad for dinner and how great it makes you feel!

If you haven't read my book, **5-Star Salad Mastery**, I do recommend doing so if you want to learn more about the power of 5-Star Salads to increase your odds of success on a raw vegan diet. But for now, let's go over the basics - the five pillars of a 5-Star Salad:

1. Include at least one pound (16 oz) of leafy greens

5-Star Salads

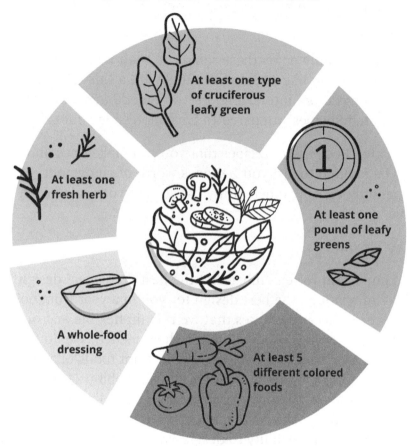

At least one type of cruciferous leafy green

At least one pound of leafy greens

At least one fresh herb

A whole-food dressing

At least 5 different colored foods

2. Include at least one type of cruciferous leafy green (kale, collards, arugula, cabbage, etc.)

3. Include at least one fresh herb (basil, cilantro, parsley, dill, etc.)

4. Include at least five different colored foods (red, orange, yellow, green, white, etc.)

5. Include a flavorful whole-food, plant-based dressing

There are several 5-Star Salad recipes in the meal plan menu that I know you will love but as you get more familiar with these 5 pillars of an amazing salad, you will have the skills and knowledge to begin creating your own 5-Star Salad recipes!

You can certainly enjoy these salads on their own as a full meal, but if you like to eat your salad with a side dish to make things more interesting, I recommend having one of the "Big Batch Recipes" prepared to have alongside your salad.

Big Batch Recipes are recipes that you can make once and it will be enough to last you 2-4 days worth of enjoyment - depending on how much of it you eat with your salad each time.

Stay Flexible

It is important to remember that the best daily meal design today may not be the best design for you in a year from now. Long-term success requires that we remain flexible and open to making intelligent adjustments when needed. We do that by utilizing a variety of healthy, whole plant foods in a way that promotes long-term health and sustainability. The Traffic Light System will help you to build a structurally sound foundation for your raw vegan diet while giving you the confidence and flexibility to design your daily meals in the best way possible for any situation.

Food Combining

Food combining is a dietary strategy which seeks to encourage optimal digestion based on the order and combination that foods are eaten. There is certainly a benefit to understanding the general concepts behind food combining, however, I do not believe in a dogmatic approach to its application.

Each person's digestive capabilities will be different based on a variety of factors such as age, activity levels, acute or chronic diseases, stress management, hydration levels, prescription and OTC drug use, antibiotic exposure, microbiome status, and so on.

I have designed the 21-Day Raw Transformation Program to naturally encourage proper food combining without you having to think about it. However, let's go over some of the main points that you should know about food combining:

1. Eat in the order of the highest water-rich foods (fruits) to the lowest water-rich foods (vegetables, nuts, seeds, avocado, salads). Water content and the general density of a food is the easiest way to know how quickly it will digest. Juicy, water-rich foods (watermelon) digest very fast - while dense, lower water-rich foods (potato) digest slower - and fatty foods (nuts) digest the slowest.

   To avoid indigestion, you want to make sure you eat the fastest digesting foods before you eat any of the slower digesting foods. This is why I have designed the *Daily Meal Design* the way that it is.

2. In general, avoid mixing fruit with any dense foods - especially cooked food. Though, some fruits in a salad (i.e.: tomatoes) are usually OK for most people. Also, blending a small amount of fruit (i.e.: dates) into a seed-based salad dressing tends to work fine for most people as well. Everyone is different, so be mindful of what works best for you.

3. Leafy greens digest well with everything.

4. Avoid drinking with meals.

5. Avoid over-eating.

6. Avoiding eating while under stress.

7. Pay attention to what digests well for you and what does not - adjust your diet accordingly.

8. Download my free food combining chart at: https://myrawintuition.com/shop/

9. I recommend reading my book, 5-Star Digestion for a deeper understanding of food combining and healthy digestion overall.

The more simple a meal is, the better it should digest. The key is finding a healthy balance between simplicity, enjoyment, nutritional adequacy, and sustainability, while optimizing digestion.

Cravings

Cravings have a bad reputation, but the truth is - a craving is just a reflection of a person's emotional and physical conditioning.

Most people have been raised in households that normalize eating high-calorie, processed foods (potato chips, pizza, and ice cream) in times of elevated states of emotions (birthdays, holidays, sporting events, etc.). So as we get older and we experience elevated levels of emotion (i.e. stress) we are emotionally conditioned to desire these types of foods.

Additionally, these highly processed foods generate a dopamine (pleasure) response that far exceeds the natural responses we get from fresh fruits and vegetables. This eventually creates a physical addiction to such foods.

Fortunately, we have the power to recondition the emotional and physical cravings that we experience. In the same way (repetition) that we trained our body and mind to desire unhealthy food, we can create new desires and attractions to healthy food.

This is a two-part solution:

1. As we mentioned earlier, we must change our level of consciousness around food so that we no longer see the typical craving foods as foods. By establishing in your mind that fast food, pizza, and cookies are not actually food - you take away any power they might have had over you.

    You can also use a visualization technique that has been successful for me: Any food that you are tempted to binge on, I want you to visualize that food in your body, breaking down into the individual chemicals or ingredients that it is made of and what they will do as they travel through your bloodstream and get incorporated into your cells. For me, this has been a very effective method for shutting down any unhealthy temptation that might arise.

    Another technique that you can use is writing a declaration on a piece of paper - for example: "I declare that from this day forward, I will not allow potato chips into my body. They contain fried, oxidized fats that are detrimental to my health and I will no longer harm myself by eating them." Then, sign your declaration.

    If you honor your word, then this should help you stop eating whatever unhealthy food that you were once tempted by.

2. Next, you must make sure that you are eating enough healthy carbohydrates to keep your body satisfied.

    There are two categories of food that you will eat in this program that should eliminate all of your cravings - fruit and 5-Star Salads!

Fruit is full of hydration, fiber, vitamins, minerals, and simple carbohydrates that your body requires to feel full and satiated. If you have a sudden hunger craving - have a few pieces of fruit and that should take care of it. Juicy fruit is ideal but you can also have a few Medjool dates - try our Chocolate Mulberry Crunch Balls on page 172. Fruit can be enjoyed throughout the day as much as needed to keep you feeling satisfied and cravings-free.

If you experience cravings for savory foods, then a mineral-rich 5-Star Salad covered in a creamy, homemade, whole-food salad dressing is the answer. These salads feature all of the heavy, loosen-your-belt, take-your-socks-off satisfaction that you need, without having to do any of those things!

Other things to consider when someone experiences cravings:

- Ensure you are staying hydrated throughout the day.

- Avoid consuming stimulants (salt, sugar, oil, caffeine, processed foods).

- Eat enough food to keep you satisfied. Under-eating leads to cravings!

- Remove all of your trigger foods from your home.

- Get enough sleep. Insufficient sleep causes hormonal imbalances that lead to cravings.

- Be intentional about building a strong, healthy microbiome with a variety of plant foods.

Where Do You Get Your _____?

Calcium: Leafy green vegetables, sprouted beans, and lentils, some fruits (citrus, dates, figs)

Protein: Leafy green vegetables, sprouted beans, and lentils, nuts, seeds, root vegetables, fruits

Iron: Leafy green vegetables, sprouted beans, and lentils, nuts, seeds, fruits

Omega 3s: Leafy green vegetables, chia seeds, flax seeds, hemp seeds, walnuts

Iodine: Sea vegetables (dulse, nori, kelp, etc.), leafy green vegetables, green beans, strawberries, cranberries, prunes, potatoes
*the iodine content of plants will vary based on the soil they are grown in.

Vitamin D: Sunlight, some mushrooms

B12: Supplementation is normally recommended

Time Saving Tips

One of the biggest concerns that I hear from people is the time commitment that it will take to eat a raw vegan diet. This is a valid concern, however there are many ways we can reduce the amount of time it takes to gather, prep, and clean up after our meals.

1. **Buy all of the produce you need for the week on the same day/trip.**
   There will of course be times where you'll need to make additional trips to the store but if you can get the bulk of what you need in one trip, it will be much more convenient for you. This may require stops at multiple

grocery stores to get everything you need but it will save you time in the long-run.

2. **Utilize Big Batch Recipes.**
   Just like batch cooking - you can make raw recipes that will last for days! There are several "big batch recipes" that you can use as sides to your dinner salad. Some of my favorites are the Hearty Vegetable Chili, Wild Rice Stuffing, Lasagna, and Pizza Bites.

3. **Mass Prepare Your Ingredients.**
   You can prepare enough salad ingredients for two or three salads at one time so all you have to do is throw everything together and enjoy! Salad dressings can last up to three days in the fridge - or up to a week if you use a vacuum blender and sealed container. So make a few batches of dressing and keep them in the fridge for faster dinner prep.

4. **Eat More Fruit.**
   Fruit is truly Nature's fast food. As I said before - you just peel it and eat it. This is why basing your breakfast and lunch meals on fruit will make life so much simpler and more efficient when it comes to food preparation and clean up.

5. **Use The Right Tools For The Job**
   One of the most effective ways to save time in the kitchen is to have the correct tools at your disposal. I've watched people try to prepare a salad with a steak knife and have a really tough time with it. So, ensure that you have a wide variety of knives, extra-large cutting boards, glass mason jars, extra-large salad bowls, a variety of glass storage containers, and whatever you feel that you will need to be successful. See my recommended kitchen tools on page 60.

Cost Saving Tips

The other common concern that I hear of eating this way is that it is too expensive. Affordability will depend upon each individual's situation, but there are various ways to reduce the cost of eating healthfully. I think it is always important to remember that healthy food might cost more today, but it will likely add up to much less than the potential hospital bills incurred due to poor health later in life. With that said, we want to make this lifestyle as affordable as possible so that it is accessible to anyone interested. So, here are a few ways to make this lifestyle more affordable.

1. **Re-evaluate Your Priorities and Mindset**
   Some people spend hundreds of dollars a month at restaurants, bars, and other forms of entertainment and don't think twice about it. But then they get a cheap frozen pizza instead of lettuce because "they are on a budget." The mindset that many people have around "what is health truly worth to me" - should be examined. What we "want" shows up in our words, but what we "believe" shows up in our actions.
   Personally, when I started to experience the health benefits of living and eating this way, I no longer desired to drink alcohol or eat poor quality food from restaurants - that saved me a lot of money! I was then able to put that extra money towards buying a higher quantity of fresh produce. So, look around at the things that you regularly spend money on (maybe things like coffee or junk foods) and see if there are any areas where you are willing to make different choices and redirect those funds to go towards healthy produce.

2. **Take Advantage of Sales**
   One thing that I always try to do is stock up on the sale items. One week navel oranges are on sale and so I buy a

lot of oranges. The next week, apples and pears are on sale, so I stock up on those. Oftentimes, different stores will be running deals on different types of produce so you can still get a good variety of produce at a reduced cost.

There are also markdown bins that offer overripe bananas and things like that, which can also help here and there.

3. **Shop at Wholesale Stores**
   If you have a wholesale store near you, such as Costco, I highly recommend taking advantage of that. This is where I get all of my frozen fruits and frozen berries, because it is so much more affordable. These types of stores also have larger containers of other fresh fruits and vegetables at a reduced cost compared to traditional grocery stores.

4. **Speak With Your Local Produce Suppliers**
   Getting to know your produce suppliers, whether that is the Produce Manager at your local grocery store or the local farmers - building a relationship with them can often lead to big savings. If you let them know that your household goes through a large amount of produce and that you would like them to keep you in mind if there are ever any discounted items or deals that come up - you would be surprised at how many deals on produce you can get.

5. **Stick To Unprocessed Food**
   One of the best ways to keep your grocery bill as low as possible is to avoid buying anything that comes in a package. Processed and packaged foods can spike a grocery bill faster than the government's attempts to steal your rights. By sticking to whole fruits and vegetables and avoiding pre-made foods, you will save big-time money.

6. **Grow Sprouts**

   Growing your food is a great way to save money in the long run. Most people, however, do not have the space or understanding of how to grow a large garden. The good news is that anyone can easily grow sprouts right on their kitchen counter for a fraction of the cost of buying these foods from the store. See the additional shopping tips below to see where you can get your own organic sprouting seeds.

Additional Shopping and Preparation Tips

* Shop at various grocery stores - including Asian Markets - to get the best deals on produce.

* Go in with family or friends on large bulk orders that you can get items at an overall discounted price and split the bill between you.

* Join a Community Supported Agriculture (CSA) group to get fresh local produce at a lower price.

* Some items such as Medjool dates can be found online (i.e.: Ebay) for a much cheaper price than you'll find at grocery stores.

* Order organic sprouting seeds at www.sproutman.com, www.trueleafmarket.com, or find them at many health food stores.

* Bananas are one of the cheapest fruits you can get. Load up on bananas and use them for smoothies, frozen nice-cream, fruit salads, etc.

* Load up on a wide variety of dried herbs and spices - these will help you create delicious recipes, so it's important to always have them on hand.

- Invest in quality kitchen appliances as much as you are financially able to.

Recommended Kitchen Tools

The tools we use can make all the difference in how we experience this lifestyle. The right kitchen tools make preparing meals easier, faster, and more enjoyable. You do not need to have the fanciest, most expensive tools available, but investing in high-quality tools and appliances for your kitchen is truly making an investment in your health.

Below are the tools that I use and recommend and where you can go to research them for yourself:

Blender

With a blender you can turn a large amount of fruits and/or vegetables into tasty smoothies, dressings, soups, sauces, and more. The nice thing about blending is that it is quick, easy, and requires minimal clean up. Blending keeps the fiber in the end product, which is beneficial for digestion, helping us feel full as well as promoting healthy bowel movements.

What I use: Vitamix 5200 (You can purchase refurbished models at a discounted price at vitamix.com). I have used it pretty much every day over the last ten years and it is still working great.

What I recommend: Vacuum blending is what I now recommend to everyone I work with. I truly believe that vacuum blending is a revolutionary way to prepare smoothies, soups, sauces, and dips. By removing the air from the container before we blend, there is a substantial reduction in oxidation of the food while blending. This equates to less nutrient loss, more antioxidants, more flavor, and smoother consistency. I have recently purchased the BioChef Vacuum Blender Container + Pump which does fit and work on my Vitamix - which is an option for current Vitamix owners. If you do not already own a Vitamix, it is worth looking into vacuum blenders at http://discountjuicers.com/blenders.html.

Juicer

Juicing fruits and vegetables separates the liquid from the fiber. This gives you a highly concentrated source of nutrients that requires very little digestive energy. Juicing requires more prep-work and clean-up than blending, but many find the extra effort to be worth it. A juicer is not required to succeed on this program, but I do enjoy juicing at times and believe that it is worth looking into if you are interested.

What I use: Omega 8006 - it has worked very well for me over the last ten years.

What I recommend: There are many newer juicers on the market today. I recommend researching the various brands at http://discountjuicers.com/juicers.html.

Food Processor

A food processor is similar to a blender but is better for slicing, shredding, and chopping - it is not for making something into a smooth consistency. I like to use the food processor for making salsas, pico de gallo, pates, mock meats, guacamole, and shredding veggies.

What I use: Breville BFP660SIL Sous Chef 12 Cup Food Processor - This food processor makes recipe creations so easy - I love it.

What I recommend: This is the food processor that I recommend to anyone in the market for a food processor. You can look more into it at https://www.breville.com/us/en/products/food-processors.html.

Dehydrator

You can use a dehydrator to make veggie chips, fruit strips, raw pizza, veggie loaves, flax crackers, dried fruits, and more! This works by removing the moisture from fruits and vegetables, allowing you to create healthy alternatives to common snack foods.

What I use: Excalibur 9 Tray - I have been using this machine for several years, and it is still working great.

What I recommend: This is the machine that I recommend to anyone in the market for a dehydrator. You can find them at https://excaliburdehydrator.com.

Water Distiller

A water distiller purifies water by duplicating nature's hydrologic cycle of evaporation, condensation and precipitation. As the water in the machine is heated, it turns to steam (leaving contaminants behind) and is then condensed and precipitates into your holding container as pure H_2O. It is the most reliable method to purify water of all of the harmful contaminants that find their way into the water supply. This includes pesticides, pharmaceutical products, industrial waste, agricultural chemicals, inorganic minerals, and much more.

What I use: The Pure Water Mini Classic CT Countertop Distiller and the AquaNui 8/5 Automatic Water Distiller - I am an affiliate for both of these distillers.

What I recommend: If you are in the market for a water distiller, you can go to https://mypurewater.com or https://myaquanui.com and use my discount code (RAWINTUITION) for 5% off of your purchase.

If you are not looking to buy a water distiller, I recommend getting a few glass gallon jugs and filling them up at a reverse osmosis water dispenser at a local grocery store. Many grocery stores are now offering this service.

Other Kitchen Essentials

• Extra-large salad bowls

• Large cutting boards

• Glass mason jars

• Chef knives and other sized knives

• Vegetable peeler

• Spiralizer and/or julienne peeler – turns veggies into spaghetti-like noodles.

These items can all be found at most kitchen retail stores or amazon.com.

Putting It Into Practice

1. **Pick your plan:** All Raw or High Raw

2. **Get clear on the foundational guidelines**

3. **Set your boundaries:** Traffic Light System + 5-Yes Test

4. **Daily meal design:** Personalize SFS

5. **Tool up for success!**

Lifestyle Basics

In addition to eating a healthy diet, how we live our lives is also a key factor in our overall health. Lifestyle is a very broad topic and there is a lot that we could cover, but the focus of this program will be on what I refer to as **The Big Three: Sleep, Stress, and Exercise.**

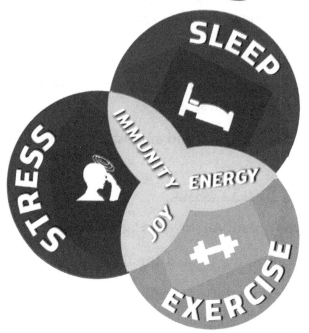

These three lifestyle factors are the basic fundamental prerequisites to creating a healthy body and mind. When in balance, they help support a parasympathetic state in the body and lead us to experience incredible improvements in immune function, energy levels, and overall joy in our lives.

This also makes it easier to stay motivated to continue making healthy food choices.

Sleep, stress, and exercise are separate components of our overall health, but they are very closely intertwined with one another. The more we improve in one of these areas, the easier it becomes to improve in all three. Likewise, the more we neglect any one of these aspects, the more difficult it will be to maintain the others.

So grab a pillow, some running shoes, and a stress ball, and let's get started:

<u>Sleep</u>

Out of "the big three," getting adequate sleep is probably the simplest one to change, but for many people it is the most difficult one to follow through with. In our modern world there are so many things that prevent or distract us from getting the sleep that we need. The good news is that we can make simple adjustments to our lifestyle, mindset, and sleeping environment that will make it easier for us to accomplish this.

In today's fast-paced world, sleep does not get the respect that it deserves when it comes to our health. Did you know that inadequate sleep can negatively alter your gut microbiome, cause hormonal imbalances, make you more likely to crave junk food, increase the risk of depression, and may lead to increased inflammation in the body?

Many people mistakenly attribute low energy levels to their diet - which certainly can be a contributing factor - but often times they are lacking energy because of the quality and duration of sleep that they are getting.

Once humanity learned to harness electricity, it became possible to remain active at all hours of the night. Since then our culture has become increasingly more insistent on working, eating, and entertaining ourselves late into the night - largely under the guise of productivity. However, does working on less sleep actually allow you to be more productive?

I often use the example of two lumberjacks (Jack and Paul) competing to chop the most wood in an hour. The competition begins and both Jack and Paul are chopping away at an equal pace. However, after 30 minutes, Jack stops for a few minutes to sharpen his axe, while Paul keeps chopping away. To the crowd, it appears as if Paul is going to win because he has now taken the lead. However, throughout the competition, Paul's axe has become dull and each whack of the axe is less effective. When Jack begins chopping again with his newly sharpened axe, he is able to chop through significantly more wood than Paul can with his dull axe. It is not long before Jack has caught up and surpassed Paul in the amount of wood he has chopped, and ultimately, Jack easily wins the competition.

I use this example to show the importance of giving your body and mind the necessary sleep to keep them sharp and effective. Pushing the body and mind to continuously work without adequate sleep will gradually reduce their performance and energy levels.

Additionally, poor quality and insufficient sleep also reduces the body's immune function and makes us more vulnerable to sickness and dis-ease. Maybe you have had the experience of coming down with a cold after several nights of poor sleep. As well, you have probably noticed that when you are sick, you tend to sleep much deeper and longer during your recovery. This is because sleep and immunity have a bidirectional relationship - meaning they both can impact the other.

During sleep, the body goes through a series of cleansing, healing, and detoxification processes. Without adequate sleep, the body cannot efficiently complete these essential functions - resulting in an accumulation of waste, and eventually, the body will display symptoms of illness.

It is similar to continually hitting "snooze" when your computer asks you to run a system update. The longer you prevent the computer from running an update and restarting, the more glitches occur in the system. Eventually, the computer will do a forced update and restart itself - just like the body initiating symptoms of acute illness (a cold or flu) to get you to rest and allow it to run its "updates" and cleanse itself.

To help the body achieve optimal energy levels and immune function it is not only important to get the proper amount of sleep, but also to provide the necessary environmental conditions that are needed to promote deep, restful sleep.

The following sleep hygiene checklist can help you evaluate your current sleep habits and make improvements if needed:

1. Be in bed by 10:00 pm at the latest (sleep and awaken as closely with the sun as possible)
2. Finish eating and drinking at least 2-3 hours before bedtime (deeper rest when there is less to digest)
3. Turn off or remove electronics from the bedroom (do not sleep next to a cell phone)
4. Make your bedroom as dark as possible (light affects melatonin production and reduces the quality of the sleep)
5. Keep the room at a cool temperature

6. Use a fan (not blowing on you) to create white noise to help you fall asleep
7. Use organic bedding if possible
8. Move the bed away from the walls to reduce exposure to dirty electricity
9. Open the window to the bedroom (if possible and safe) to allow fresh air into the room before or while you sleep
10. Avoid stimulants (food, drinks, drugs, etc.) - especially in the afternoon

Stress

If there is one thing that can sabotage a person's health faster than a poor diet, it would be chronic stress. A little bit of stress can be helpful to push us out of our comfort zone and help us evolve physically, mentally, and spiritually. However, when stress is suppressed and is not allowed to be released from the body or mind - it becomes chronic and can erode the foundation of a person's health and steal the joy from their life.

Types of stress:

Eustress (good stress): The stress we experience during a challenging workout, completing an important project, or taking someone on a date. Think of things that give you "butterflies" in your stomach. This stress can be beneficial to our overall well-being and fuel our motivation and sense of purpose in life.

Distress (bad stress): The stress we experience from a perceived threat or danger. This type can be debilitating and often give us a feeling of panic or despair. Examples that could cause distress are the loss of a job, receiving an unwanted medical diagnosis, or being chased by an angry dog.

Acute Stress (short term): This is stress that we experience only for a short time and then we can recover and return to a state of homeostasis. This can be in the form of either eustress or distress - such as giving a presentation (eustress) or escaping from the angry dog (distress).

Chronic Stress (long term): This is stress that we experience for extended periods of time and are not able to recover from fully. Chronic stress can lead to persistent low-grade inflammation, which can weaken the immune system, negatively alter the gut microbiome, and contribute to hormonal imbalance and depression. Some causative factors that are associated with chronic stress are: living under oppressive governments, living in a dysfunctional household, abusive relationships, or the continued mental or physical pain associated with a chronic illness.

Identifying, Processing, and Releasing Stress

We all experience stress throughout our lives but it is how we *perceive* that stress and how we react to it that will determine its impact on us. You may have noticed that two people can react to the same situation in very different ways. For example, two people who receive the same medical diagnosis of having a degenerative chronic disease can have two completely different perceptions of their situation.
The first person views the diagnosis as devastatingly bad luck and spends the next twelve months being depressed, eating junk food, complaining that life is unfair, and continues to have declining health. The other person sees the diagnosis as a wake up call and an opportunity to improve the way that they live their life. They change their diet and lifestyle, start exercising, and spend more time in nature - and twelve

months later, they feel like a brand new person and are told by their doctor that they are in remission. These two people experienced the same stressful event, but their perception and reaction to the event created different outcomes.

The way in which we handle stress as adults is subconsciously programmed into us as young children. We tend to react to stress in a way that is very similar to how we witnessed our parents react when they were stressed. This can be a good thing or a bad thing - depending on how we were programmed.

It is essential to become aware of how you respond to stress in your life. This will help you identify if your habitual perceptions and reactions serve you or sabotage you. Once you gain this awareness you can learn to implement healthier ways of processing and releasing stress - so that it does not become chronic.

Three general questions to ask yourself to help you determine if you handle stress effectively:

1. Do you perceive the situation through an <u>optimistic lens</u> (as an opportunity for personal growth) or through a <u>pessimistic lens</u> (as a punishment from the universe)?
2. Do you approach the situation as a <u>creator</u> of your reality or a <u>victim</u> of your circumstances?
3. Do you hold in or try to <u>suppress</u> stress and tension in your body or do you find healthy outlets to process and <u>release</u> the emotions that you feel?

Everyone is different and should process stress in whatever way works best for them - but with that said, I believe the following steps can help anyone work through stress in a healthy way:

- Identifying the source of stress
- Determine the lens you are choosing to see the situation through (optimism vs pessimism)
- Establish the role that you play in finding a solution (creator vs victim)
- Utilize healthy outlets to process the emotion (release vs suppress)

There are many outlets that can be helpful with processing stress in our lives:

- Exercise
- Spend time in nature
- Talk with someone you trust
- Journal
- Creative expression
- Breathwork
- Meditation
- Hot bath with epsom salt and essential oils
- Laugh
- Allowing yourself to cry
- Spend time with a companion animal
- Get a massage
- Volunteer / Help others in need
- Join a community group

Maintaining Balance

Ideally, we want the majority of the stress that we encounter to be eustress and a minimal amount to be in the form of distress. Of course, life happens and we just have to do the best that we can in each situation.

By maintaining healthy levels of eustress and distress (with the tips above) and effectively processing them as they acutely come up - this will help to prevent the formation of chronic stress - allowing us to support a healthy immune system and increase the joy we experience in our life.

Exercise

The human body was made to move! Society has increasingly become more sedentary as technology and modern conveniences have advanced. Even among health-conscious individuals, like raw vegans - it is incorrectly assumed that eating a healthy diet lessens the need to partake in exercise.

Unfortunately, many people believe that the main purpose of exercise is weight loss - but this is not true. Independent of diet, exercise improves the health of our gut-microbiome, supports the lymphatic system, improves mitochondria function, benefits mood, and so much more! So even if you eat healthy and are maintaining a healthy weight, you should still be exercising regularly if you want to optimize your mood, energy levels and overall long-term health.

When we exercise, we tell the body that we need to be better and more efficient at producing energy, which stimulates an increase in the body's capacity for mitochondrial biogenesis (creating more mitochondria throughout the body). Mitochondria are energy producing organelles within our cells that produce cellular energy called adenosine triphosphate (ATP).

Think of ATP as gasoline for the engine of our cells. If our population of mitochondria is not healthy enough to produce sufficient "gasoline" for our cells to function, we will experience fatigue and low energy. This makes it critical for our lifestyle habits to support the proper creation and strengthening of the mitochondria in our cells.

Mitochondria are especially susceptible to high levels of oxidative stress, so regular moderate exercise in combination with a healthy, colorful, antioxidant-rich diet is crucial to stimulating the creation (and protection) of new, healthy mitochondria throughout the body.

In addition to promoting healthy mitochondria, exercise is strongly linked to improved mood and mental health. I am sure you have experienced that blissful feeling after a good workout. With exercise, we improve blood flow, stimulate lymphatic circulation to aid with detoxification, and generate beneficial hormones, such as BDNF and endorphins.

There are various forms of exercise that we can choose to incorporate into our lifestyle that will provide us with these benefits:

HIIT (High-Intensity Interval Training) - Periods of intense exercise separated by periods of recovery. This is a popular style of exercise with exceptional mitochondrial benefits. **Strength/Resistance Exercise** - weight lifting, resistance bands, yard work, pushups, sit-ups, pull-ups, squats, lunges, hill walking, biking, stair climbing, etc.

Endurance Exercise - running, jogging, biking, hiking, brisk walking, jumping jacks, etc.

The best type of exercise is the one that you will regularly do - so find one or more types of exercise that you enjoy and make it part of your routine. Ideally, 3-5 times per week is a good target to aim for and you can always do more if desired.

As with any new exercise routine, start slow and build up your intensity as you can.

Putting It Into Practice

The perfect complement to your healthy diet is a healthy lifestyle. Some of the main takeaways I want to highlight from this section are:

1. Sleep plays an important role in supporting the immune system and maintaining optimal energy levels. Get to sleep early and create an environment for deep, uninterrupted sleep.
2. Effective stress management is essential for supporting the immune system as well as promoting a joyful outlook on life. Identify any sources of stress that you have and how you currently manage it. Then, work on finding healthy ways to process and release it, if needed.
3. Regular exercise goes beyond weight loss. It is required for optimal energy levels, as well as maintaining emotional and mental health. Find one or more exercises you enjoy and make it part of your regular routine.

Detoxification Optimization

So far in this program, we have covered the "what, why, when, and how" of eating. But when it comes to creating a healthy and sustainable diet and lifestyle - what we consume is only half of the equation. Many people overlook the vital importance of supporting the body's ability to eliminate the waste products that are generated from daily living. In this section, we will focus on some important steps we can take to help the body efficiently carry out its natural detoxification processes.

To better appreciate how the body detoxifies itself, it is helpful to have a basic understanding of how the body works:

To put it simply, the human body is composed of a bunch (trillions) of cells and two main fluids – blood and lymph. Each cell has a specific job to do in the body – think of them as trillions of microscopic people living in the community of your body, all working together for a common cause. Just like you and me, each one of these cells requires a source of nutrition (food) for their energy and a way to eliminate their waste products in a hygienic way (a bathroom with working plumbing and sewage systems).

As we eat food, the body begins the process of digestion by breaking the food down into its smallest parts, then absorbs the nutrients through the intestines, which then make their way into the bloodstream. Think of your bloodstream as the kitchen of your body, delivering the nutrients that your cells need to survive and do their work. After the cells have been fed, they need a place to "go to the bathroom" and dispose of their waste products – this is where your lymphatic system comes in.

The lymphatic system is essentially your body's sewer system that collects cellular waste products and carries them to the lymph nodes (akin to septic tanks) to be rendered down into a more manageable substance, and then carried to the eliminative organs to be removed from the body. Think of the lymphatic system as the waste management department of the body, where the "garbagemen" work. These garbagemen are working all day, every day, continually visiting each person (cell) in the community and collecting their trash.

Imagine if the waste management services could not keep up with your community's demands, and rather than stopping at your house once every week, they came once every month. At the same time, imagine if your plumbing stopped working and you could not flush your toilets. As you can imagine, trash and waste would start to pile up, creating a toxic environment, attracting all sorts of bacteria, flies, rodents, and so on. It would not take long before sickness and disease began to manifest in anyone living in this environment.

Throughout history, malnutrition and poor waste management systems have been underlying causes of disease in communities around the world – and the same can be said for the cellular communities within the human body. Cellular waste is acidic and must be removed in a timely manner, or inflammation and damage to the cells will ensue. Just like the person living in a home without a working toilet – a cell with no way to remove its waste products will eventually become sick. So, for the health and wellbeing of our cellular communities, we must maintain healthy fluids.

Keeping the fluids and tissues of the body healthy

Let's start with a very basic chemistry lesson that can help us understand acidity versus alkalinity and what that means for the fluids and cells of the body. We measure the level of acidity or alkalinity using the pH scale. This scale ranges from

0 (most acidic) to 14 (most alkaline), with seven being neutral. Foods like fresh fruits and vegetables are rich in alkaline minerals (calcium, potassium, magnesium, and sodium) and generally have an alkaline influence on the body. Other foods, such as meat, dairy, and eggs (higher in sulfates, chlorides, phosphates, and organic acids), will generally have an acidic influence on the body.

Alkalinity promotes an internal environment that is cooling, flexible, and anti-inflammatory. In contrast, high acid levels in the body create an environment that is corrosive, rigid, and pro-inflammatory. When conditions in the body become too acidic, the body becomes stiff and dehydrated, joints become sore, and tissue damage can occur. For this reason, it is vital for the long-term health and longevity of the human body to practice a diet and lifestyle that encourages a predominately alkaline environment within its fluids and tissues.

The pH level of our blood must remain within a very narrow range (between 7.35 and 7.45) for us to survive. Thankfully, the body regulates blood pH for us automatically, although our diet and lifestyle greatly affect the amount of effort the body must exert to do so. When someone consumes a diet comprised predominantly of alkaline-forming foods (fruits and vegetables), the body efficiently maintains the proper blood pH without any trouble.

However, when someone consumes a diet rich in acid-forming foods (animal products and processed foods), this quickly increases the amount of acids entering the bloodstream, and the body must take immediate action to keep the blood from becoming too acidic – a condition known as diet-induced metabolic acidosis. One way the body does this is by increasing the activity of cells called osteoclasts, which release calcium from the bones to neutralize the acidity in the blood. While this process helps to avoid a crisis in the short-term, over time, the bones and connective tissue may become weak, kidney stones may form, and other inflammation related conditions could occur if this cycle continues.

Additional methods that the body may use to combat an acidic environment is by producing more cholesterol (an anti-inflammatory lipid), or by concentrating water to the affected area (seen as edema).

The long-term effects of overly acidic diets, especially those high in animal fat and protein, may increase our risk of:

- Heart disease, blood clots, and stroke

- Cancer

- Kidney disease

- Dementia and Alzheimer's

- Osteoporosis

- Depression

It should be clear that we are best designed to consume a diet that supports a predominantly alkaline internal environment without, "robbing Peter to pay Paul." Creating an imbalance in one part of the body in order to bring balance to another part is not a sustainable model of health. Lucky for us, the perfect matrix of fiber, antioxidants, hydration, vitamins, minerals, polyphenols, amino acids, fatty acids, and other phytonutrients contained in whole plant foods allows the body to maintain homeostasis (balance) in all of its systems harmoniously.

When the fluids of the body are healthy, they flow elegantly like a winding river, circulating and supporting all of the various cells and tissues. However, when we consume a diet high in fat, we quickly see a thickening of our body's two main rivers – blood and lymph. Within just hours of eating a high-fat meal, we can see an increased viscosity (thickness) of these fluids and reduced function and flexibility of blood.

To make matters worse, diets high in saturated fats negatively alter the gut microbiota and intestinal permeability, allowing harmful components to enter the bloodstream that lead to oxidative stress and inflammation – like releasing a swarm of angry bees into your blood vessels and making the body's immune cells wade through molasses while trying to catch and remove them.

Imagine in your mind that you have come across a small river running through a pristine forest. The current is flowing smoothly, and the water is so clear that you can see straight to the bottom. You bend down and cup some of the clean, cool water into your hand and take a sip to refresh yourself before continuing on your journey. Now imagine coming back to this same location one week later to find that several sizable trees have fallen into the river, severely restricting the flow of the current and creating large areas of stagnant water. Within these stagnant areas, the water has become murky, and algae has developed on the surface. Mosquitoes and other microbes have inhabited the area, and an unpleasant smell permeates the air. You, nor any other animal, would be safe to drink the water in this stagnant condition - just as the cells in our body are not safe to function in fluids that are stagnant and murky from too much fat in the diet.

Eating high amounts of fat (especially animal fat) is like dropping trees throughout the body's rivers (circulatory system), leading to increased viscosity of the fluids and plaque accumulation on the vessel walls. In this condition, it is more difficult for the fluids to properly nourish the cells and delays removing their waste. The longer there is stagnation, the more toxic the environment becomes.

Instead, when we fill our bodies with fresh fruits and vegetables, it is like taking a fiber-made chainsaw and cutting through the dams that have formed, releasing the stagnant fluids. The two main rivers of the body are once again able to flow freely and support a healthy environment for the trillions of cells that make up the human body.

Pathways of Elimination

To complete this basic overview of the body, it is vital to understand the importance of elimination.

If you only remember one thing, let it be - *what you don't eliminate, you accumulate* - meaning, if we do not effectively remove cellular and metabolic waste, as well as the ever-increasing environmental pollutants from our bodies, we will accumulate more toxins than the body can safely handle – and health problems will arise.

As mentioned above, the lymphatic system is an essential partner to the eliminative organs, working hand-in-hand to efficiently remove toxic waste from the body. Unfortunately, on top of a poor diet, the sedentary lifestyle that many people engage in today undermines their lymphatic system's ability to do its job efficiently. The good news is that we can make changes to our diet and lifestyle that will support the lymphatic system and promote healthy elimination.

- **Daily movement** – Physical activity stimulates the circulation of our lymphatic fluid. Schedule a few five to ten-minute walks each day or walk up and down some stairs to get your circulation moving. Develop the habit of doing some pushups, jumping jacks, or some other form of exercise each day. Avoid sitting for long periods by setting daily reminders on your phone to get up and move. A lifestyle that promotes regular movement is essential for a healthy lymphatic system.

- **Breath fully** – The diaphragm and lungs are as close to a pump as we have for the lymphatic system. The motion of full, diaphragmatic, nasal breathing helps to stimulate the circulation of lymphatic fluid.

  Most people breathe fast and shallowly from their mouth into their chest, leading to poor gas exchange in the lungs and insufficient movement of the diaphragm muscle. Nasal breathing encourages us to breathe deeper into the stomach, engaging the diaphragm to expand and contract. Breathe slowly through the nose, into the belly, and exhale completely.

- **Avoid using lotions and creams on the skin** – The skin is the body's largest eliminative organ. Most health and beauty products that are applied to the skin will clog the pores and impede the elimination of toxins and waste products from the body. Although the skin is water-proof, it is also very absorbent to many chemicals.

  Most lotions and creams contribute MORE toxins into the body as they absorb through the skin and enter the bloodstream. The golden rule to remember with health and beauty products is: **If you would not eat it, do not put it on your skin!**

- **Dry skin brush daily** – One of my favorite lymphatic tools is the dry skin brush. Using a dry, natural, stiff-bristled brush to gently but firmly exfoliate the skin, we can remove dead skins cells while increasing blood and lymphatic circulation. For directions on how to perform this technique, see The Daybreak Detox Support Routine on page 96.

- **Sweat often** – The best way to cleanse the skin and keep it healthy is to sweat often. The skin is our largest eliminative organ and provides a pathway for the elimination of toxins, such as carbon dioxide and heavy metals. The detoxifying function of the skin plays a vital role in the regulation of the body's overall toxic load.

  In today's culture, many people undermine their skin's detoxification efforts with antiperspirants, lotions, creams, colognes, perfumes, tight synthetic clothing, air conditioning, and bathing in chemical-laden water. Instead, support skin health and detoxification by avoiding toxic "beauty" products, filter your bath water, wear clothes made of natural fibers, and sweat often through physical activity, sun exposure, or saunas.

- **Get enough sun** – Appropriate sun exposure increases immunity, boosts mood, and is great for the whole body, including the skin. Sun exposure prompts the body to produce important hormones, such as vitamin D, and also encourages detoxification through the pores.

  It is important to avoid repeated sun-burns, as this can cause damage to the skin and increase the risk of skin cancer. The best way to protect the skin from burning is to use clothing to cover the skin or to move into shade, rather than using synthetic chemical lotions.

- **Drink pure water** – Hydration is essential for the health of both blood and lymphatic fluid. A diet of fresh fruits and vegetables is hydrating on its own, so you may not feel thirsty as often as you would eating cooked food. In addition to the hydration from diet, I drink as much distilled water as I need to stay properly hydrated (see my recommended home distillers on page 62).

This usually includes 32 ounces to start my day and up to 32 ounces in the afternoon. Everyone's hydration needs will vary, so adjust as needed. I recommend drinking distilled or reverse osmosis water. In almost all cases, I would avoid using tap water for drinking and cooking.

- **Avoid eating animal fat and animal protein** – As previously mentioned, these items introduce additional toxicity (environmental pollutants, endotoxins, etc.) into the body while increasing fluid viscosity, reducing circulation, and compromising the pathways of elimination.

- **Eat a whole-food, fiber rich, plant-based diet** – Fiber, antioxidants, hydration, electrolytes, and vitamins promote a smooth flowing lymphatic system while simultaneously supporting the organs of elimination.

Now that you know how to optimize the efficiency of your lymphatic system, we need to put on our "OSHA (Occupational Safety and Health Administration) hats" and ensure we are keeping the body's exits clear of obstructions. There are five main exits or pathways of elimination to keep up to code:

Kidneys

The kidneys are two bean-shaped organs that sit at the back of the abdominal cavity, one on each side of the spine. The kidneys perform many functions including regulating fluid levels, blood pressure, and electrolyte balance, as well as filtering and removing waste products by way of the urine.

Diet and lifestyle factors play an important role in supporting kidney health. Consuming foods rich in animal protein can increase the acid load in the blood and cause hyper-filtration of the kidneys, causing inflammation and impairment to kidney cells.

Additionally, high-fat foods, especially those containing saturated fat and trans-fat, can reduce the kidney's ability to filter waste from the blood. The kidneys are highly vascular organs, and just like any other part of our vascular system, they can become clogged with fatty deposits, decreasing their function.

How to support the kidneys:

- **Eat an antioxidant-rich, low fat, whole food, plant-based diet**: Plant proteins (and fats) have <u>not</u> been shown to cause the same damaging effects to the kidneys that animal sources have. In fact, polyphenol compounds in fruits and vegetables have been shown to have protective effects on kidney cells, reduce renal inflammation, and improve kidney function.

- **Hydration**: Adequate hydration is essential for maintaining proper kidney health. When the body is consistently in a dehydrated state, there is an increased risk of kidney stone formation and injury to the kidneys. Without proper hydration, the various waste products that are filtered through the kidneys become increasingly more concentrated, which can strain and inflame the kidneys. As hydration increases to appropriate levels, we see a dilution of these waste products, making it easier and safer for the kidneys to filter them out of the body.

I encourage you to drink water that is free from as many inorganic minerals and pollutants as possible. Distilled water and reverse osmosis water are, therefore, my top choices for drinking.

- **Stay active**: Sedentary lifestyle habits are associated with impaired kidney function. Both the amount of time spent being physically active and the amount of time spent being sedentary have independent effects on the heath and function of the kidneys.

  More physical activity is associated with more favorable kidney function and less kidney damage, while more sedentary behavior is associated with poorer kidney function and more kidney damage. Regular uninterrupted periods of sedentary behavior of 30 minutes or longer may worsen kidney function.

  In essence, the more active we can be, the better off our kidneys will function. So, move more and sit less. Set regular 30-minute reminders to get up and move your body if you commonly sit for long periods.

Colon

The colon is the final five to six feet of the intestinal tract, where food spends the longest amount of time on its journey through the digestive system. While food makes its way through the colon, trillions of bacteria break down fiber and other components into metabolites that can have various biological effects within the gut and throughout the body.

It is the colon's job, with the help of commensal (beneficial) bacteria, to absorb the beneficial components passing through it and to eliminate everything else through the stool in a timely manner. If the foods we eat spend too much time in the intestines (i.e. constipation) they begin to ferment and putrefy, releasing harmful degradation byproducts that damage the intestinal lining and cause inflammation in the body.

On the other hand, when food moves too quickly through the intestines (i.e. diarrhea), there is not enough time to sufficiently break down and absorb what we need. Ideally, we should see a bowel transit time (how long it takes for food to travel from mouth to anus) of roughly eighteen to twenty-four hours. You can test this yourself by eating some organic corn or a large helping of beets and timing how long it takes for you to see it come out the other end.

The body also uses the colon to eliminate excess hormones, cholesterol, heavy metals, and other inorganic substances. This makes our bowel-transit time especially important, as we want to have as little contact between these substances and our gut lining as possible to avoid irritating the tissue. Additionally, if our elimination is too slow, there is an increased risk of reabsorbing some of these toxins that the body is attempting to remove.

The health of our colon largely depends on maintaining a proper bowel transit time and there are several ways we can help to achieve this:

- **Fiber is your colon's best friend**: A variety of fiber is what helps to produce a healthy population of good bacteria in the colon. A healthy balance of bacteria in the gut encourages good gut motility and the steady movement of food through the system. Fiber also binds to excess bile, heavy metals, and other toxins and carries them out of the body through the stool. With a fiber-rich diet, we promote healthy bowel movements that move through the colon at the proper pace.

- **Hydration is essential:** This may surprise you, but a healthy sample of stool should be comprised of about seventy-five percent water! Water increases the bulk of stool, which helps it to stimulate the gut wall to move through the intestines at an appropriate pace. One function of the colon is to absorb water from the stool as it makes its way towards the exit. As stool loses its water content, the harder it becomes, and the slower it moves through the colon. Hard stool can be difficult and painful to pass. So, it is essential to drink enough clean water and eat plenty of fresh, water-rich fruits and vegetables to add bulk and hydration to the stool and prevent constipation.

- **Avoid stress at mealtime:** Stress can wreak havoc on digestion and bowel transit time. During times of stress, we activate the sympathetic nervous system, and the body goes into "fight or flight" mode. This diverts the body's attention away from tasks like digestion and sends blood and energy resources to the muscles in our arms and legs. Even if there is no immediate threat to our safety, we can still trigger this stress response by merely thinking stressful thoughts. Before you eat, take a moment to clear your mind, take a few slow, deep breathes into your abdomen, and settle into a state of peace and gratitude.

- **Movement:** Regular physical activity contributes to a healthy bowel transit time. Even something as simple as a light walk before or after a meal can help to encourage proper intestinal motility and elimination.

- **Do not hold it in:** The act of intentionally delaying a bowel movement is one of the most harmful behaviors someone can commit against their colon. This keeps stool inside the colon longer than necessary and exposes the intestinal wall to prolonged contact with harmful waste products. The longer a bowel movement is delayed, the higher the risk of reabsorbing toxins becomes. The moment that we feel an urge to pass a bowel movement, we should honor the body's signals and find a bathroom as soon as possible.

Lungs

The lungs are two large, spongy organs located in the chest that allow us to breathe in vital elements from the atmosphere, such as oxygen, nitrogen, and carbon to be used in biological processes. These organs also function as an eliminative pathway to release metabolic waste products such as carbon dioxide and heat as we exhale. Only a thin, single-celled membrane separates the air in the lungs from the blood stream. It is vital that we keep these delicate organs healthy and do what we can to optimize our breathing environment.

- **No smoking**: This may seem obvious, but I am not only referring to cigarettes. People smoke a variety of different plants with the belief that they confer a health benefit. While some plants may be safer to smoke than conventional tobacco, any time something is burned, it generates various harmful gases and particulates, such as partially oxidized hydrocarbons and polycyclic aromatic hydrocarbons, that can cause cellular damage. Avoiding breathing smoke of any kind to protect long-term health of the lungs. I recommend finding alternative methods of consuming medicinal elements.

- **Cruciferous vegetables:** The phytochemical, sulforaphane, found in cruciferous vegetables has been shown to stimulate phase II enzymes that protect epithelial cells in the lungs from inflammatory air pollutants. By eating a diet high in antioxidant-rich fruits and vegetables, especially cruciferous vegetables (broccoli, cauliflower, kale, arugula), we can help to support the body's ability to limit damage to the lungs from environmental assaults, such as air pollution.

- **Optimize your indoor air quality:**

    o Plants are not only good to have in your diet, but in your home as well! Indoor plants brighten up a room and can help to purify certain contaminants from your indoor living space.

    Toxic gases, such as volatile organic compounds (VOCs) and aldehydes, are emitted from many household materials such as paint, wood preservatives, furnishings, printers, glues, permanent markers, aerosol sprays, chemical cleaners, disinfectants, air fresheners, dry-cleaned clothing, pesticides, and more.

    Common toxic gases, like formaldehyde and ethylbenzene were shown to be reduced from indoor air by 50% and 75%, respectively, after indoor plants were introduced. If you have pets, you will want to research the best plants to have in your home, as some plants can be toxic to dogs and cats.

    o Maintain good ventilation in your home. Open windows when possible.

    o Use non-toxic household products, including paints, bedding, cleaning supplies, air fresheners, personal care products, etc.

- ○ Consider using a good quality air purifying machine.

- **Diaphragmatic nasal breath work** – Relax your neck and shoulders while in a seated or reclined position. Place your hands lightly on your belly and breathe in slowly through your nose. Feel your hands rise as the air fills your stomach. Now, breathe out slowly through the nose until the air leaves your stomach. Continue slow diaphragmatic nasal breathing for three to five minutes or as long as desired. This is a great exercise to practice in the morning and before going to bed.

  Nasal breathing can increase nitric oxide levels in the body and may help to reduce inflammation and relax the tissues in the lungs. Additionally, the nasal mucosa functions to trap pathogens and prevents potentially harmful particles from reaching the lungs in the first place. Regularly breathing through the nose encourages a parasympathetic (rest and digest) state in the body, which can reduce inflammation and relax the muscles in the airways.

Skin

You may not think of your skin as an organ, but it is, in fact, the largest organ of the body. The skin functions as a barrier to the outside world but has many other responsibilities such as regulating body temperature, receiving stimuli from the environment, nutrient storage, and eliminating waste products.

The skin is equipped with millions of tiny openings, called pores, that allow the skin to release oils, sweat, and other waste products. The oils secreted through the pores moisturize the skin, repel water, regulate the skin's pH, and maintain a healthy skin microbiome. Washing the skin too often, especially with commercial cleaning products, strips the skin of its natural oils and can cause dehydration and cracking to occur. It is best to simply use clean water to wash the skin and if needed, a non-toxic, chemical-free soap, as minimally as possible.

Sweat plays a key role in maintaining skin health as well. When we sweat, the pores secrete water, electrolytes (such as sodium), and various proteins that protect the skin from environmental pathogens. Additionally, sweat acts as a means of transport for eliminating metabolic waste products and environmentally acquired pollutants, such as ammonia, urea, arsenic, cadmium, lead, mercury, bisphenol A (BPA) and other environmental toxins. This makes the skin another vitally important detoxication pathway that must be respected and cared for.

More ways to support your skin:

- **Eat the rainbow**: We are exposed to a variety of stressors (UV radiation, environmental pollutants, poor diet, etc.) that can lead to oxidative stress and inflammation of the skin. Consuming a wide variety of colorful pigments in our diet provides the skin with an ample supply of antioxidants to combat oxidative damage. A colorful diet is, in essence, a natural form of sunscreen that provides a level of full-spectrum protection from inside out.

- **Get adequate sunshine:** Appropriate sun exposure on as much of the skin as possible, offers several health benefits including immune system enhancement, hormonal regulation, and detoxification support. This makes direct sun exposure (without the use of sunscreen) an essential part of maintaining a high level of health. Sunscreens commonly contain toxic chemicals that inhibit the skin from adequately synthesizing vitamin D. I believe that the residues that coat the skin from commercial soaps and detergents also have impeding effects on the skin's ability to utilize sunshine. Instead of using toxic products from companies that put their profits above our health and safety, we can simply put on additional clothing, wear a hat, seek shade, or go indoors when we have had enough sun exposure.

- **Sweat:** As mentioned above, sweating is a vital detoxification function that the body uses to eliminate waste products and environmental toxins. Sweat flushes out the pores and maintains an open channel of elimination.

  Avoid the use of antiperspirants and other synthetically made personal hygiene products. The chemicals contained in these products are absorbed through the skin and increase the body's toxic load. At the same time, these products clog the pores and obstruct the skin from eliminating the waste that is already inside.

- **Dry skin brush:** The skin is continually shedding thousands of old cells each day and dry skin brushing helps to clear some of those dead cells from the surface of the skin. This allows for more efficient detoxification of waste products through the skin and also encourages lymphatic flow throughout the body. Five minutes of brushing in the morning or before going to bed is a great way to improve the condition and function of the skin.

- **Avoid harmful chemicals:** We encounter harmful chemicals in essentially every aspect of our lives these days and many of them can damage the integrity of the skin. This includes makeup, soaps, shampoos, detergents, lotions, hair spray, nail polish, perfumes, colognes, lawn chemicals, pesticides, bug sprays, and even the water we drink and bathe in.

Harmful chemicals do not only get into the body through what we eat, but also by what we drink, breath, and put on our skin. The body was not designed to encounter such a heavy and consistent chemical assault, so it is vitally important to avoid these synthetic chemicals as much as possible to maintain the health of our skin and overall well-being.

Nasal Mucosa

The nasal mucosa lines the nasal cavity from the nostrils to the pharynx. It functions to capture allergens, dust, and pathogens that enter through the nose and then facilitates an immune response to neutralize and eliminate these particles from the body. When this happens, an increase in mucous production is initiated, often resulting in a "runny nose."

In addition to the mucus lining, various hairs throughout the nasal cavity help to filter and eliminate pathogens. Larger hairs near the nostrils catch dust, pollen, and other pathogens and keep them from possibly getting into the lungs. Further back in the mucosa are additional tiny hairs, called cilia. These microscopic hairs work in unison to rhythmically sweep the mucus that has captured airborne invaders to the back of the throat to be coughed out through the mouth or swallowed and eliminated through the digestive tract.

On top of that, we produce an endogenous gas in the paranasal cavities called nitric oxide that has antibacterial properties and also modulates the rhythmic flow of the ciliary hairs. It is like having a constant mist of antibiotics being sprayed in the nasal passage that only harms pathogenic microbes while providing benefits to the healthy cells.

As you can see, the nasal cavity and mucosa have various methods of defense to keep the body free of pathogens. Here are a few ways we can support the health and function of this gateway into the body:

- **Stay hydrated**: The body produces about 1.5 liters of mucous daily to protect the body from infection, keep tissues hydrated, and remove toxins from the body. Mucous is mainly composed of water, so keeping the body hydrated helps it to produce sufficient mucous when you need it the most.

- **Embrace the nose hair**: As previously mentioned, nose hair acts as a barrier to foreign particles in the air we breathe. Trimming a few hairs that find their way out of the nostrils is no problem but refrain from going too far and trimming hairs further within the nostrils. Removing too many nose hairs can increase the risk of air pollutants getting past the nasal cavity and into the lungs.

- **Avoid intranasal drugs, if possible**: Various popular drugs that are applied directly into the nose for conditions such as allergic rhinitis can have harmful effects on the nasal cilia, reducing their ability to clear mucous from the nasal cavity. This allows irritants to remain in the nasal cavity longer than we would like and increases their potential to cause harm. Consider natural alternatives, such as a neti pot or essential oils.

- **Blow that nose**: A simple way to ease the burden on the nasal cavity is to gently blow the nose. I often see individuals sniffing mucous back up into their nose rather than using tissue and eliminating what the body is trying to remove. Instead of using one-time-use tissues, designate a few old t-shirts to repurpose as reusable hankies and use them to blow your nose into.

- **Optimize nitric oxide:** We can increase our body's production and circulation of nitric oxide by eating more nitrate-rich leafy green vegetables, eating polyphenol-rich fruits and vegetables, maintaining a low-fat diet, breathing through the nose rather than through the mouth, and even by simply humming your favorite song for a few minutes.

Putting It Into Practice

When all five eliminative pathways are supported and cared for, we optimize the body's ability to reduce its toxic load and focus its energy on healing and health maintenance. To experience the highest levels of health, the body must be able to efficiently eliminate its waste products faster than they can accumulate.

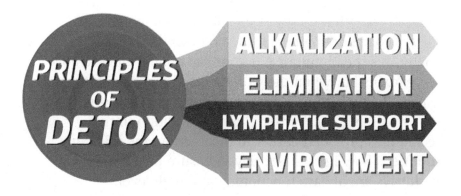

Detoxification is a natural function of the body; however, the rate at which the body is able to detoxify itself depends largely on how we care for it. To encapsulate what we have covered in this section and to highlight the steps we can take to support the body's detoxification efforts, I have laid out the four foundational principles of detoxification for you to implement in your life.

Principle #1: Alkalization (Diet and Hydration)

As we have covered in this section, diet and hydration play key roles in maintaining the proper pH levels throughout the body. When we alkalize the tissues and fluids of the body with fresh fruits and vegetables, we nourish the cells while creating a catabolic environment that helps to dissolve obstructions that may have accumulated throughout the body. Additionally, proper hydration levels allow the body to mobilize waste products to the eliminative pathways to be removed from the body. This is the first step towards creating fluidity and balance within the body.

Principle #2: Eliminative Pathway Optimization

As the effects of an alkalizing diet begin to energize the body and mobilize accumulated toxins, the second principle of detoxification is to optimize the eliminative pathways. The organs of elimination must be able to handle the increased load of toxins trying to exit the body. Under normal conditions the eliminative organs can comfortably remove daily toxins but when the workload suddenly increases, it is especially important to give extra support to our organs so that we do not overburden them. In addition to the techniques provided earlier in this section, the following routine is how I start each day to ensure my eliminative pathways are always functioning at a high level.

The Daybreak Detox Support Routine

1. **Get to bed early**: Yes, this routine starts the night before. A good seven to eight hours of restful sleep is one of the best ways to ensure I will have the energy

and motivation to stick to my daybreak routine. Ideally, I try to be in bed no later than 10:00 pm and wake no later than 6:00 am. The later I go to bed, the less rejuvenated I feel when I wake up the next day, so it is important to me that I adhere to an early bedtime.

It is also important to create a sleep oasis for yourself that supports the deepest levels of sleep possible – remove electronics from the room, turn off the wi-fi, put the phone in another room, avoid looking at screens an hour before bedtime, make the room completely dark, and keep the temperature slightly cool.

A critical factor that has a significant role in determining sleep quality is whether you breathe through your nose or through your mouth during sleep. Mouth-breathing during sleep can increase the risk of dis-ordered breathing patterns, such as sleep apnea, that prevent us from reaching the deep, restorative levels of sleep we need.

Breathing through the nose filters, conditions, and warms the air we breathe, keeping the airways moist and allows for air to distribute throughout the lungs easier. Make it a habit to blow your nose before bed to ensure you have a clear nasal airway and can breathe through your nose throughout the night. If needed, look into getting mouth tape to help you with nasal breathing during sleep.

2. **Clean out the pipes:** The first thing I do upon waking each day is visit the bathroom and release the waste and toxins that my body gathered for elimination over the night. A healthy body should initiate a bowel movement and urination shortly after waking up for the day. The longer waste is retained in the body, the

more toxins potentially get reabsorbed back into the body and the higher our toxic load becomes. By "cleaning out the pipes" first thing after waking, we set the body up for success in its efforts to maintain a clean and healthy internal environment.

This includes the "upper pipes" as well – I gently blow my nose each morning (and as-needed throughout the day) to clear out any excess mucous that may have accumulated over the night. I used to be one of those people that would ignore a runny or congested nose, continuously sniffling throughout the day – do not be one of those people. You might be surprised at how much of a difference it can make in how clear-headed you feel during the day by proactively blowing your nose at the first sign of excess mucous or congestion in the nasal cavity. Clean "pipes" make for a clear mind.

3. **Open the pores**: Next, I spend about five minutes dry skin brushing my whole body to exfoliate dead skin cells, open up my pores, and stimulate blood and lymph circulation. Any dry, natural, stiff-bristled brush can be used. There are many ways to do this, but I start at my head, face, and neck, working with short, moderately firm, brush strokes downward towards my heart. Then, I do the same on my arms and legs, working from my hands and feet, inward to the heart. As I move down the neck and inward from the arms and legs, I make sure to brush over the lymph nodes (in the neck, armpits, and groin) a couple times with the intent of improved lymphatic flow. I finish with a few large clockwise (from my point of view looking down) circular brush strokes over my stomach, tracing over the colon.

Skin brushing is an invigorating way to start each day that primes the lymphatic system by promoting healthy circulation, opening the pores, and allowing the skin to better support the body's detoxification efforts.

4. **Loosen up**: With my lymphatic system primed, I like to do five to ten minutes of light stretching to warm up my muscles, work out any tension, and further support optimal circulation throughout my body. I believe flexibility is an important component of longevity for both the body and mind. Having good range of motion in our joints help us to maintain optimal mobility and agility throughout life. I find stretching to be a great way to connect with my body, while helping me focus on the present moment and get into a powerful state of mind.

5. **Flush the system**: Now that the pipes are clean and the exits are open, I hydrate and "flush out" my system with about 32 ounces of purified water. I personally choose to drink steam <u>distilled water</u>, as I find it to be the most reliable way to avoid the ever-increasing environmental pollutants that collect in our water supply and can cause devastating long-term harm to our health. An important aspect of helping the body to detoxify effectively is to decrease, as much as possible, the amount of toxins we expose ourselves to every day – and clean water is a vital part of that.

6. **Connect with the breath**: When I am ready, I find a comfortable place to sit in complete silence, connecting with my breath, breathing through my nose as I settle into a meditative state. Nasal breathing activates the parasympathetic nervous system and makes it easier to relax and release any built-up tension that I may be holding in my body or mind.

As I sit comfortably, I will do an alternate nostril

breathing exercise, breathe holds, or some other type of nasal breathing exercise, or simply just sit quietly and enjoy the silence as I gently breathe in and out of my nose and connect with my breathe. The point is to begin each day in a composed and focused state and at the same time, build nasal breathing habits that improve the efficiency and function of the breath.

7. **Sweat it out** – The final phase of my routine is to break a sweat through some form of exercise. This is typically done through one or more of the following: push-ups, pull-ups, dumbbell exercises, squats, sit-ups, planks, jogging, running, rebounding, or climbing stairs. By working up a sweat, I not only help my body to detoxify itself, but also promote better brain and cardiovascular function throughout the rest of the day. I commit to getting at least 30 to 45 minutes of exercise before I start each day.

This is the basic routine that works well for me, and it is one that I have developed to be sustainable for my lifestyle. Many people attempt to implement a routine that is too difficult or complicated to maintain and after a couple weeks they have given up on it.

The key is to arrange your home and environment in such a way that it makes whatever change you are working to achieve, as easy and convenient as possible. For example, each night I set a full container of water and my skin brush on the bathroom counter, so that they are ready for me to use the next day. If I had to go to the kitchen and fill up my water container, or search for my skin brush, I would probably skip those steps more often and I would never build the momentum to solidify this routine into a lasting habit.

By consistently following the Daybreak Detox Support Routine, I have experienced more sustained energy, focus, and productivity throughout my days. I believe having a positive routine to begin each day is one of the most powerful ways to be successful in anything you are trying to achieve. The first few hours after waking up are powerful for programming the subconscious mind and setting the tone for the rest of the day. Whether you choose to follow the routine outlined above or one of your own, I encourage you to start your days with intention and direction and your life will begin to change.

Principle #3: Lymphatic Support

With the body alkalized, toxins mobilized, and the eliminative pathways wide open, it is vital to support the healthy flow of lymphatic fluid. As previously mentioned, the lymphatic fluid is the vehicle that collects toxins and carries them to the eliminative organs to be removed from the body. There are many techniques to support the function of the lymphatic system that have already been mentioned but just to reiterate a few of my favorites:

- Dry skin brush

- Rebounding

- Running/jogging/speed walking

- Diaphragmatic breathing

- Massage

- Low-fat, plant based diet

- Adequate hydration

Principle #4: Environmental Awareness

Implementing the first three principles of detoxification can go a long way towards significantly enhancing the health of our body and mind. The fourth principle of detoxification augments the effectiveness of the other three principles by reducing the overall toxic load that the body needs to deal with going forward. It would be counterproductive to put in the effort of enhancing the body's detoxification potential if we are going to turn around and reintroduce the same toxins back into the body.

Becoming keenly aware of our environment is vital in the pursuit of optimal health and well-being. In our current environment, toxic chemicals are ubiquitous, and we must do our best to reduce our exposure as much as possible.

Avoid as much as possible: tap water, pesticides, lawn chemicals, indoor air pollutants, animal fats, pharmaceutical products, dental products, most personal care products, thermal paper receipts, electromagnetic radiation, heavy metals, etc.

In the world today, it has become increasingly necessary to make detoxification the foundation of one's lifestyle. This does **not** mean that we should perpetually put the body through intense cleanses or fasts. However, we must do our best to create an internal and external environment that supports the body's natural detoxification processes. The chemicals in many of the products mentioned above disrupt the body's endocrine system, leading to hormonal problems that result in various common diseases.

It would be wise to boycott the companies and products that are making us sick and work towards creating a safer, cleaner environment for ourselves and future generations. Support local, organic farmers, environmentally conscious companies, ethical small businesses, grow your own food – including sprouting and microgreens. It is up to us to be (and support) the change we want to see in the world, and I believe we start by recovering our health, living consciously, and educating others to do the same.

Support Systems

The final pillar that will make your transition to a raw vegan diet and lifestyle successful is the support systems that you set up around yourself. They say *if you want to go fast, go alone - but if you want to go far, go together*. By surrounding yourself with a strong group of supportive people and resources, you can create an environment that makes it impossible to fail.

Early in my raw vegan journey, I attended two certification programs (The Graff Academy of Raw Food Education and The International School of Detoxification), where I met other like-minded people who shared the same passion and enthusiasm for health that I did.

These were two of the most memorable and life-changing experiences that I have ever had, and the supportive relationships that grew out of them were incredible. After each of these events, we formed online groups to stay connected and support each other and this was invaluable to me on my journey.

Over the years, I have continued to meet many new, inspiring people - both in-person and online - that continually help to reinvigorate my passion for the raw vegan lifestyle and healthy living. There is a positive, synergistic effect when you surround yourself with high-vibrational people.

Building strong support systems is necessary for everyone - but it is especially important for anyone that feels alone on their raw vegan journey, or finds that this new lifestyle clashes with their current social circle. I am telling you right now - this experience and your results can be infinitely better when you put yourself in the right environment.

Gaining Awareness

As with everything else - to create change, we must first gain a deeper awareness of our current situation.

- Evaluate how your current relationships (online and in-person) and interactions make you feel: Do they energize you and leave you feeling inspired? Or do they drain you and leave you feeling frustrated?

- Also, consider if the people you spend time around (online or in-person) help to expand your knowledge or skills in any way. As Les Brown says, "If you are the smartest person in your group, you need to find a new group!"

- Take a piece of paper and draw a line vertically down the middle. On the left side, list all the people and relationships that energize or inspire you. On the right side, list all the people and relationships that drain you. Be honest - nobody else needs to see this list but you.

It is critical to have a clear picture of your social environments - both in-person and online.

Adjust and Prioritize

Now that we have more awareness of the social environment that we are in, we can make adjustments and prioritize those that have positive influences in our lives.

- Determine which relationships add positivity and personal growth to your life and spend more time building those relationships. You do not need to completely disassociate with those people that tend to drain your energy, but especially in the beginning of your journey, it can be helpful to limit those interactions.

- You do not need to tell someone that they drain you or that they make you feel bad about yourself. Many times, this can be a close friend or family member that you do not want to hurt their feelings - so if they ask why you haven't been around as much, just let them know that you are working on some personal things and are taking time for yourself.

- This list can change over time. You may want to rearrange which relationships you prioritize as you, and others around you, change.

Build Connections

It is up to you to build the best "team" of positive people around you. The most successful companies recruit the best talent to help them achieve their goals - in the same way, you should be proactively looking to build connections with other people that are doing the things that you want to be doing and that you can learn from.

- Write down a list of 3-5 people or organizations (online or in-person) that you find inspiring and would like to emulate in some way.

- Study their actions and discover how they learned to do what they do.

- Reach out and see if there are any opportunities to work with them to build a better relationship.

- Join groups (online or in-person) where you can meet new people and create a new network of positive people.

We tend to become like the people that we hang around the most. If you surround yourself with quality people that inspire and encourage you to be the best version of yourself, then your level of success will exponentially increase.

This principle also applies to the media that we consume, the music we listen to, and the books we read, and anything else the puts a message in our mind.

Throughout my journey, I have consistently consumed motivational and educational content, and interacted with positive people. We must proactively build a positive environment for our minds to manifest a positive reality.

Build Your Confidence

At the end of the day, *you* need to be your biggest supporter of all. The world will see you how you see you. So the level of confidence that you have in yourself will be the nucleus that attracts everything and everyone else to you.

Remember to take time to be with yourself as well. Sometimes spending time alone - away from the opinions of others - is the best way to hear our genuine thoughts and desires.

And as you continue to educate yourself and gain experience with this lifestyle, your confidence will grow, and you will naturally be less affected by other people's reactions to your choices.

If you are like me, and you have a deep intuitive knowing that this lifestyle is what you have been called to do - then I encourage you to step into your power and follow your heart. Have a clear understanding of *why* you want to live this way and go for it.

Remember that you don't light a candle in a well-lit room, so if others do not understand why you want to live this way, that is OK. Be an example of health and live your truth with integrity.

Putting It Into Practice

1. Gain awareness of your current social environments.

2. Adjust and prioritize your relationships to support your success.

3. Proactively build your social circle by recruiting new, positive people and networks.

4. Solidify your confidence and resilience.

Designing Your Shopping List

Staple Items To Always Have On Hand

- **Bananas** (fresh and frozen): Consider buying by the case
- **Dates:** I recommend buying in bulk from farms (online) or from wholesale distributors
- **Fresh fruit:** It's important to always have an ongoing rotation of seasonal, fresh fruit
- **Frozen fruits**: Mango, blueberry, strawberry, etc. (if you have a Costco near you, they have the best prices I have found on frozen fruits and berries)
- **Dried herbs and spices**: Basil, cayenne, Cajun, chili flakes, chili powder, chipotle, chives, cinnamon, cumin, curry, dill, garlic granules, onion granules, oregano, paprika (regular and smoked), pumpkin spice, rosemary, sage, taco seasoning, thyme, turmeric
- **Specialty items that may need to be ordered online**: Frontier Pizza Seasoning, Kirkland's No Salt 21 Seasoning, garam masala seasoning, mesquite powder, nori sheets, dulse flakes, maca powder

Buying Your Greens

At the beginning of each week, you will need to buy at least (7) Base Greens, (4) Supplemental Greens, and (4) Fresh Herbs. You can select any combination of the greens from each category to get the amounts needed.

The size of the head or bundle of greens will vary, so if your grocery store only has small heads of lettuce, you may need to buy a few extra heads or bundles so that your salads are big enough each day.

You can buy boxed or bagged, pre-washed greens when needed - to save time on preparation - but I do recommend buying as much of your greens as individual heads as you can if they are available.

To help you remember to rotate your greens, I recommend purchasing whatever greens are on sale each week. Since sale and discounted items usually rotate, this will help you to switch up the greens that you are eating over time - plus it saves you money!

Rotating the greens you eat each week will help you consume a wider variety of different nutrients and diverse types of fiber.

Base Greens (x7)
Iceberg
Romaine
Spinach
Spring Mix
Butter Lettuce
Green Leaf Lettuce
Red Leaf Lettuce

Supplemental Greens (x4)
Arugula (3 oz box)
Beet Greens
Bok Choy
Baby Bok Choy
Cabbage
Chard
Collards
Dandelion Greens
Endive
Kale
Mustard Greens
Radicchio

Fresh Herbs (x4)
Basil
Cilantro
Dill
MInt
Parsley

Buying Your Vegetables

Vegetables really brighten up a salad with their various vibrant colors. The goal for your weekly shopping trip is to get enough vegetables to add at least five different colors (including the green from the leafy greens) to each one of your 5-Star Salads throughout the week.

Each color represents a different phytonutrient (antioxidants, polyphenols, etc.) that will support a healthy gut microbiome.

Example:
Carrots (orange)
Onions (purple)
Tomatoes (red)
Summer Squash (yellow)
Leafy Greens (green)

The example above would give you 5 different colors to fill your daily salads with throughout the week - just make sure you pick up enough of each ingredient to last you for each day of the week you are shopping for.

Asparagus
Beets (only organic)
Bell Peppers
Broccoli

Carrots
Cauliflower
Celery
Corn (only organic)
Cucumber
Fennel
Garlic
Ginger
Jalapeño
Leek
Mushrooms
Okra
Onions
Sprouts
Summer Squash
Tomatoes
Watercress
Zucchini

<u>Buying Your Fruits</u>

When it comes to buying fresh fruits, the variety will vary greatly, depending on the season. It is best to eat as locally-grown and in-season as possible, but do not let the proximity of where fruit is grown to deter you from enjoying a wide selection of delicious, nourishing varieties.

Bananas, for example, are a perfect staple fruit for most people to rely on year-round. They are inexpensive, versatile, and calorie-dense. I always make sure I have a large stash of bananas in the kitchen to use for smoothies, nice cream, and snacks.

I have found that other tropical fruits like mango, papaya, and pineapple are usually the most affordable from Asian Markets or wholesale suppliers (such as Costco).

The best deals on berries are most often going to be in the frozen section rather than fresh. Again, wholesale suppliers are usually the most economical option for buying berries.

Dates are another calorie-dense fruit that can be especially helpful for extinguishing cravings that may come up, particularly at the beginning of your transformation. You can often find dates in bulk amounts, online, directly from the farms at discounted prices.

Each season has its own notable staple fruits that you can lean on throughout the year:

Spring Staple Fruits
Mango
Pineapple
Kiwi
Apricots
Bananas
Berries

Summer Staple Fruits
Nectarines
Plums
Cherries
Peaches
Berries
Bananas
Mango
Melons
Papaya

Autumn Staple Fruits
Apples
Figs
Grapes
Bananas
Papaya
Pomegranates
Persimmons
Pears

Winter Staple Fruits
Apples
Citrus
Dates
Bananas
Pears

Whichever fruits you are buying for the week, you must make sure you have more than enough. If we run out of fruit, we lose a significant source of calories - and when we are low on calories, we are susceptible to cravings and making less than optimal food choices.

In the first couple weeks, you may need to make an additional trip to the store (to restock your fruit stash) at the beginning of your transformation as you learn how much fruit it takes to last you for a week - this will be different for everyone.

An example of my weekly (winter) shopping trip is something like this (buying for 2 - 3 people):

20 bunches of bananas (a typical bunch has about 6 bananas)

15-20 pounds of citrus (navel oranges, cara cara, etc.)

On average, I will buy (1) 10 - 11 lb. box of Medjool dates (online) every other month.

Roughly 10 - 15 apples (any variety)

About once a month I go to a wholesale warehouse (Costco) and stock up on organic frozen fruits: (3) 5lb. bags of mango, (2) 4lb. bags of blueberries, (2) 4lb. bags of cherries

Use these amounts as a guide for yourself but do not feel obligated to duplicate what I have listed above.

You will get more comfortable over time with your understanding of how much fruit to buy each week. Soon it will be effortless for you to know how much to buy each week/month.

21 Day Raw Vegan Meal Plan

This 21-day meal plan will guide you through three weeks of eating a raw or high-raw vegan diet - depending on which path you choose. Each day you will be given suggested recipes for breakfast, lunch, and dinner - which will follow the basic outline of SFS (smoothie, fruit, salad).

You are also provided with 15 "big-batch sides" that can be paired with any dinner salad. These recipes are intended to ease your transition and deliver that extra bit of satisfaction while you get accustomed to eating bigger salads for dinner. Each big-batch recipe should provide about three days worth of enjoyment. If, for any reason, you cannot make one of the suggested big-batch sides, then choose another side from the list to replace it with (if a side is desired). Remember that the salad should always be the main dinner meal.

If you choose the high-raw path, you can add a side of steamed vegetables, potatoes, soup, or other consciously cooked whole food to supplement your dinner salad. Consciously cooked foods should only be eaten with your dinner salad as your last meal of the day. Consciously cooked foods should always be used as a supplement and should not displace your regular raw dinner salad. At Myrawintuition.com, you will find a downloadable addendum to this meal plan that contains various "Raw Intuition Approved" consciously cooked recipes that you can use to supplement your raw dinner salads.

For snacks, you are provided five simple and delicious recipes, but your goal should be to choose fresh fruit for snacking as much as possible. Dehydration and undereating are often contributing factors to snack cravings - so consume enough juicy fruit to keep yourself satisfied and hydrated.

The recipes listed for each day are only suggestions, so if you especially like certain recipes and want to repeat those recipes more often, feel free to do so. I do that myself - I find a few recipes that I really like, and I make them frequently. Over time, the specific recipes that I am drawn to will change and so I am always just listening to my body. It is all about following your intuition, staying flexible, and having fun with the process.

This meal plan is designed to be as simple and practical as possible; however, it will still require a significant amount of effort and patience - remember the three Ps! I want you to approach the next three weeks with the understanding that eating healthy and making big salads every day is not always fun (it can be!), but it is definitely worth it. Keep in mind that the longer you practice any new activity, the easier it gets - so stay persistent.

Get excited about reconnecting with your food and putting positive energy into the meals you eat. This is your opportunity to take control of your health and move powerfully in the direction of the life you deserve. Nobody can do the work for you. If you are serious about reaching your health and lifestyle goals, then it is time to take the action that is necessary to do so. You either make results, or you make excuses. At the end of the day, you are worth however much effort it requires for you to become confident eating this way - and I know you will be grateful that you made this commitment to yourself.

Your new life begins today!

Day 1

Breakfast

Banana Mango Bash

5 - 10 ripe bananas

1 - 2 cups frozen mango

1 - 2 cups spinach

1 - 2 tsp chia, flax, or hemp seeds (optional)

1 - 2 cups purified water, or to desired consistency

Add all of the ingredients into your blender.

Blend until smooth.

Enjoy!

Lunch

Seasonal fruits of choice, for example:

Spring: 2 mangoes & 1/2 of a pineapple

Summer: bowl of 2 chopped nectarines & 3 sliced bananas

Autumn: 3 apples & 4 figs

Winter: bowl of 2 chopped apples, 1 chopped pear, 1 banana, & handful of mulberries

Dinner

Smokehouse Salad

1 medium to large head of romaine lettuce, chopped

1 - 2 cups kale, finely chopped

1/4 cup cilantro, chopped

2 carrots, shredded or chopped cup red onion, chopped

7 - 10 grape tomatoes, whole or sliced

2 stalks celery, chopped

Add all ingredients to a large salad bowl and mix well.

Day 1, cont'd.

Smokehouse Dressing
3 Tbsp sunflower seeds
2 Medjool dates, pitted
1/2 lemon, peeled
1 clove garlic
1 tsp dijon mustard
1/2 tsp chili pepper flakes
1 tsp smoked paprika
3/4 cup purified water

Add all ingredients to a blender and blend until smooth.
Pour over your salad and enjoy!

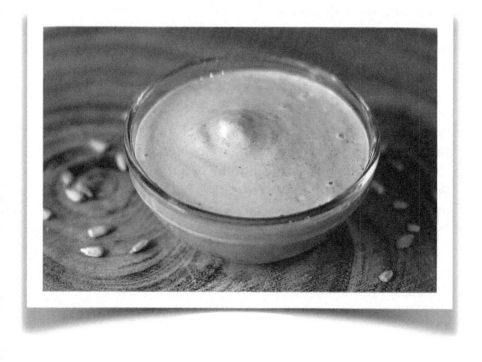

Day 1, cont'd.

Suggested Big Batch Side
Raw Vegan Vegetable Chili
Makes 3 large servings - enjoy 1 serving (this equals a volume
of around 2 soup bowls) and save the rest for Days 2 and 3.

Base ingredients:
7 Roma tomatoes
1 cup sun-dried tomatoes, soaked in water for at least 1 hour
1 cup of the soak water
1/2 cup walnuts, soaked in water for 4 - 8 hours then rinsed
1 stalk celery
1 clove garlic
1/3 cup yellow onion
1/2 jalapeño (remove the seeds, if desired)
2 Medjool dates, pitted
1 medium red bell pepper
2 Tbsp thyme
2 Tbsp sweet basil
1 Tbsp chili powder
1 Tbsp cumin

Add all of the base ingredients together in a blender, placing
the most water-rich ingredients in the blender first (closest to
the blade) and blend until smooth.
Pour into a large mixing bowl and set aside until the chunky
ingredients are ready.

Chunky ingredients:
2 medium zucchini, chopped
1 medium cucumber, chopped

Day 1, cont'd.

4 stalks celery, chopped
3 medium carrots, shredded
5 Roma tomatoes, chopped
1 cup sweet peas
1 cup corn (optional)

Use a food processor to chop (with the S-blade) the zucchini, cucumber, celery, and tomatoes, separately.
Add your chopped ingredients to the mixing bowl that the base mixture is in and mix well.
Use the shredding blade to shred the carrots.
Add the shredded carrots to the mixing bowl.
Add the sweet peas and corn (optional) to the mixing bowl.
Mix everything together very well.
Serve and enjoy.

If desired, place the final mixture in a dehydrator set at 118 degrees Fahrenheit for up to a couple of hours to give it a slightly warmer feel.

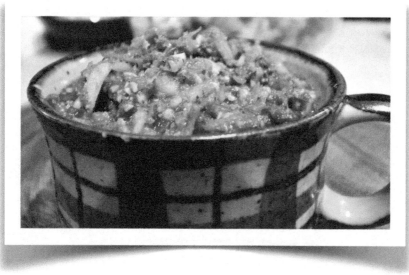

Day 2

Breakfast

<u>Blueberry Basil Elation</u>
5 - 10 ripe bananas
1 - 2 cups frozen blueberries
1 cup kale, chopped
1/4 cup fresh basil
1 - 2 tsp chia, flax, or hemp seeds (optional)
1 - 2 cups purified water, or to desired consistency

Add all of the ingredients into your blender.
Blend until smooth.
Enjoy!

Lunch

<u>Seasonal fruits of choice</u>, for example:
Spring: bowl of 3 chopped peaches & blueberries
Summer: 1 honeydew or cantaloupe melon
Autumn: 1 papaya
Winter: 3 pears & 2 apples

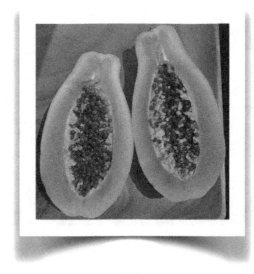

Day 2, cont'd.

Dinner

Supreme Taco Salad

1 medium to large green leaf lettuce, chopped
1 - 2 cups kale, chopped
1/2 - 1 cup button mushrooms, chopped or sliced
1/2 cup frozen corn, thawed
1/4 cup red onion, chopped
1/3 cup red bell pepper, chopped
1/4 cup cilantro, chopped
2 carrots, shredded or chopped
7 - 10 grape tomatoes, whole or sliced

Add all ingredients to a large salad bowl and mix well.

Taco Supreme Dressing

3 tbsp white sesame seeds
2 Medjool dates
1/4 cup red bell pepper
1 clove garlic
1/2 lemon, peeled
1 tsp Frontier taco seasoning
1/2 tsp paprika
1/8 tsp cayenne
3/4 cup purified water

Add all ingredients to a blender and blend until smooth.
Pour over your salad and enjoy!

Suggested Big Batch Side

Raw Vegan Vegetable Chili

Enjoy serving #2 of 3 of your leftovers.
Warm in the dehydrator at 118 degrees Fahrenheit for up to a
couple of hours to give it a slightly warmer feel.

Day 3

Breakfast
Maca Mango Sunrise
5 - 10 ripe bananas
1 - 2 cups frozen mango
2 - 3 Medjool dates
2 tsp maca powder
1 - 2 tsp chia, flax, or hemp seeds (optional)
1 - 2 cups purified water, or to desired consistency

Add all of the ingredients into your blender.
Blend until smooth.
Enjoy!

Lunch
Seasonal fruits of choice, for example:
Spring: 3 kiwis & 1/2 of a pineapple
Summer: 3 mangoes & handful of strawberries
Autumn: large bowl of grapes & 3 figs
Winter: 6 oranges & dried mango slices

Dinner
Brazilian Maca Salad
1 medium to large head romaine lettuce, chopped
1 - 2 cups kale, finely chopped
1/4 cup cilantro, chopped
2 carrots, shredded or chopped
1/4 cup red onion, chopped
1/2 - 1 cup frozen green peas, thawed
7 - 10 grape tomatoes, whole or sliced

Add all ingredients to a large salad bowl and mix well.

Day 3, cont'd.

Brazilian Maca Dressing
3 Tbsp Brazil nuts (almonds can be substituted)
2 dates, pitted
1 clove garlic
1/2 lemon, peeled
1 heaping tsp Maca
1 tsp onion granules
1 cup purified water

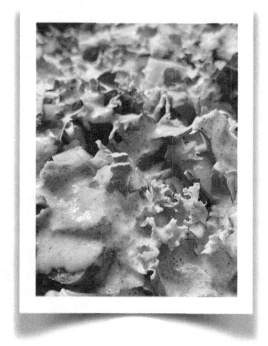

Add all ingredients to
a blender and blend
until smooth.

Pour over your salad
and enjoy!

Suggested Big Batch Side
Raw Vegan Vegetable Chili
Enjoy final serving of your leftovers.

Warm in the dehydrator at 118 degrees Fahrenheit for up to a
couple of hours to give it a slightly warmer feel.

Day 4

Breakfast
<u>Berry Celebration</u>
5 - 10 ripe bananas
1 - 2 cups frozen blueberries
2 stalks celery
2 - 3 Medjool dates
1 - 2 tsp chia, flax, or hemp seeds (optional)
1 - 2 cups purified water, or to desired consistency

Add all of the
ingredients into
your blender.

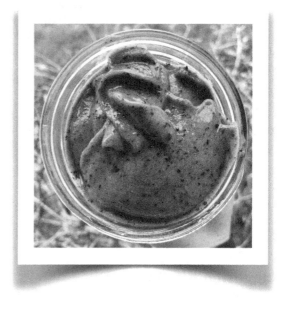

Blend until
smooth.

Enjoy!

Lunch
<u>Seasonal fruits of choice</u>, for example:
Spring: 3 apricots & 3 mangoes
Summer: 4 peaches & handful of cherries
Autumn: 4 persimmons & 2 apples
Winter: bowl of 3 sliced bananas mixed with handful of dried
mulberries & cinnamon

Day 4, cont'd.

Dinner

Creamy Italian Salad

1 medium to large head green leaf lettuce, chopped
1 - 2 cups kale, finely chopped
1/4 cup basil, chopped
1/4 cup red onion, chopped
2 carrots, shredded or chopped
1/2 medium cucumber, chopped
7 - 10 grape tomatoes, whole or sliced

Add all ingredients to a large salad bowl and mix well.

Creamy Italian Dressing

3 Tbsp sunflower seeds
1/2 lemon, peeled
2 Medjool dates, pitted
1 tsp onion granules
2 tsp Frontier Pizza Seasoning
3/4 cup purified water

Add all ingredients to a blender and blend until smooth.
Pour over your salad and enjoy!

Suggested Big Batch Side

Tuno Sliders

Makes 4 servings - enjoy 4 to 5 sliders and save the rest for
Days 5 and 6.

1 - 2 cucumbers
2 large carrots
3 stalks celery
1/2 cup sunflower seeds, soaked for 4 - 8 hours then rinsed

Day 4, cont'd.

1/2 cup almonds, soaked for 8 hours then rinsed
1/2 cup yellow onion, chopped
Juice of 1 lemon
1/4 cup parsley, chopped
2 tsp dulse flakes
2 medjool dates, soaked in water for 1 hour
1 heaping tsp yellow mustard

Add all ingredients (except the cucumbers) to a food
processor and process until thoroughly combined.
Cut the cucumbers into slices.
Top each cucumber slice with a generous amount of tuno
salad.
Serve and enjoy!
Store leftover tuno salad in a glass container in the fridge for
up to 5 days.

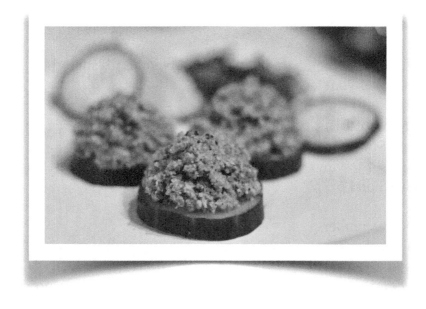

Day 5

Breakfast

<u>Cinnamon Sweet Surprise</u>
5 - 10 ripe bananas
4 - 5 Medjool dates
1/4 tsp cinnamon
1 - 2 cups purified water (or to desired consistency)

Add all of the ingredients into your blender.
Blend until smooth.
Enjoy!

Lunch

<u>Seasonal fruits of choice</u>, for example:
Spring: bowl of 3 sliced bananas, strawberries, & blueberries
Summer: 1 papaya
Autumn: large bowl of grapes & 3 figs
Winter: 4 apples, handful of dates, & celery sticks

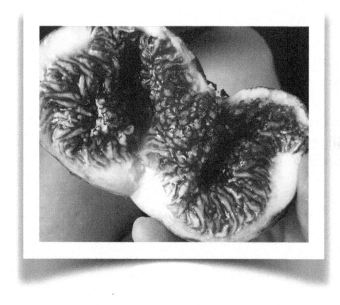

Day 5, cont'd.

Dinner
Spicy Thai Almond Salad
1 medium to large head of romaine lettuce, chopped
1 - 2 cups kale, finely chopped
1/4 cup cilantro, chopped
1/4 cup red onion, chopped
1/2 cup frozen corn, thawed
2 carrots, shredded or chopped
7 - 10 grape tomatoes, whole or sliced

Spicy Thai Almond Sauce
3 Tbsp almonds
1/2 lemon
1/4 inch ginger
2 dates
1 tsp pepper flakes
1 tsp garlic granules
1 tsp organic miso
1/4 tsp paprika
3/4 cup water

Add all ingredients to a blender and blend until smooth.
Pour over your salad and enjoy!

Suggested Big Batch Side
Tuno Sliders
Enjoy serving #2 of 3 of your leftovers.

Day 6

Breakfast

<u>Blueberry Mango Gratification</u>
5 - 10 ripe bananas
1 cup frozen blueberries
1 cup frozen mango
1/4 cup cilantro
1 - 2 tsp chia, flax, or hemp seeds (optional)
1 - 2 cups purified water, or to desired consistency

Add all of the ingredients into your blender.
Blend until smooth.
Enjoy!

Lunch

<u>Seasonal fruits of choice</u>, for example:
Spring: bowl of 2 chopped mango & 2 sliced bananas
Summer: 5 plums & a bowl of cherries
Autumn: 2 pomegranates & a large bowl of grapes
Winter: 3 pears & a few dates

Dinner

<u>Dillicious Salad</u>
1/2 medium to large head green leaf lettuce, chopped
2 cups spinach, chopped
1 cup kale, finely chopped
1/4 cup cilantro, chopped
1/2 cucumber, chopped
1/4 cup red onion, chopped
1/2 - 1 cup frozen peas, thawed
2 carrots, shredded or chopped
7 - 10 grape tomatoes, whole or sliced

Add all ingredients to a large salad bowl and mix well.

Day 6, cont'd.

<u>Dillicious Dressing</u>
3 Tbsp Sesame Seeds
1/2 lemon, peeled
2 Medjool dates, pitted
1 clove garlic
1 tsp onion granules
1 heaping tsp dijon mustard
1 heaping tsp dried dill
3/4 cup purified water

Add all ingredients to a blender and blend until smooth.
Pour over your salad and enjoy!

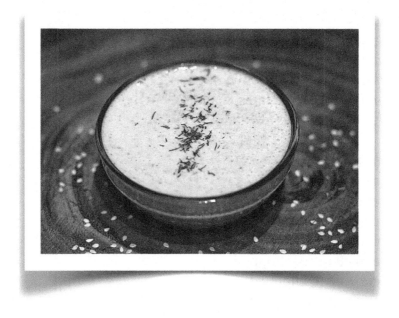

Suggested Big Batch Side
<u>Tuno Sliders</u>
Enjoy final serving of your leftovers.

Day 7

Breakfast
Berry Chocolate Dream
5 - 10 ripe bananas
2 - 3 Medjool dates
1 - 2 cups frozen blueberries
2 tsp carob powder
1 - 2 tsp chia, flax, or hemp seeds (optional)
1 - 2 cups purified water, or to desired consistency

Add all of the ingredients into your blender.
Blend until smooth.
Enjoy!

Lunch
Seasonal fruits of choice, for example:
Spring: 3 kiwi & 2 bananas
Summer: 1 watermelon
Autumn: 3 figs & 3 bananas
Winter: 3 apples & 3 oranges

Dinner
Blazin' Cajun Salad
1/2 large head green leaf lettuce, chopped
2 cups spinach, chopped
1 cup kale, finely chopped
1/4 cup basil, chopped
1/3 cup red bell pepper, chopped
1/4 cup red onion, chopped
2 carrots, shredded or chopped
7 - 10 grape tomatoes, whole or sliced

Add all ingredients to a large salad bowl and mix well.

Day 7, cont'd.

<u>Blazin' Cajun Dressing</u>
3 Tbsp sunflower seeds
2 Medjool dates, pitted
1/2 lemon, peeled
1 clove garlic
1 tsp onion granules
1/2 tsp cajun seasoning
1/2 tsp paprika
1/4 tsp turmeric powder
3/4 cup purified water

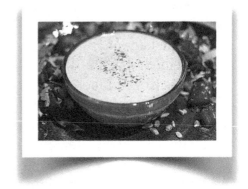

Add all ingredients to a blender and blend until smooth.
Pour over your salad and enjoy!

Suggested Big Batch Side
<u>Zughetti and Meatless Balls</u>
Makes 3 servings - enjoy 1 serving and save the rest for Days
8 and 9.

Components:
5 large zucchini
1 cup of Raw Marinara Sauce
3 Tbsp Raw Walnut Meat
2 - 3 button mushrooms, thinly sliced and chopped

Making the Zughetti Noodles:
Use a spiralizer or a julienne peeler to turn your 5 zucchini
into noodles - peel the skin from the zucchini before
spiralizing.
Place your zughetti noodles in a mixing bowl.

Raw Marinara Sauce:

Day 7, cont'd.

1 ½ cups grape tomatoes or 5 Roma tomatoes
1/2 cup sun-dried tomatoes, soaked in water for 1 hour
3 Medjool dates, pitted
2 tsp onion granules
2 Tbsp apple cider vinegar
2 Tbsp Frontier Pizza Seasoning

Add all ingredients to a blender and blend until smooth.
Add 1 cup of Marinara Sauce to the mixing bowl.

Raw Walnut Meat:
3/4 cup walnuts, soaked in water for 4 - 8 hours then rinsed
3/4 cup sunflower seeds, soaked in water for 4 - 8 hours
3/4 cup sun-dried tomatoes, soaked in water for at least 1
hour then rinsed
1 cup sweet onion, chopped
1/2 cup parsley, chopped
2 tsp thyme
2 tsp sage
2 tsp paprika
2 tsp chili powder
1 clove garlic

Place all ingredients (except the chopped parsley) into a food
processor with the "s-blade" and process until thoroughly
combined.
Add the chopped parsley and pulse until it is well combined
with the rest of the mixture.
Add 1 - 3 Tbsp of Walnut Meat to the mixing bowl.

Add the thinly sliced and chopped mushrooms.

Day 7, cont'd.

Mix well until everything is thoroughly combined.
Serve and enjoy!

If desired, place the final mixture in a dehydrator set at 105 degrees Fahrenheit for 1 - 2 hours to soften the noodles and give it a more traditional pasta mouth-feel. You can also omit the Raw Walnut Meat for a fat free version of this recipe.

Store leftovers in glass containers in the fridge for up to 5 days.

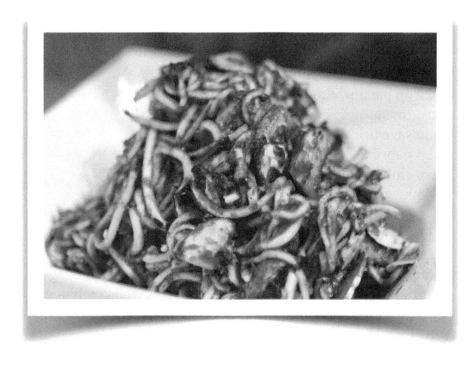

Day 8

Breakfast
<u>Cherry Maca Delight</u>
5 - 10 ripe bananas
1 - 2 cups frozen cherries
2 tsp maca powder
1 - 2 tsp chia, flax, or hemp seeds
1 - 2 cups purified water, or to desired consistency

Add all of the ingredients into your blender.
Blend until smooth.
Enjoy!

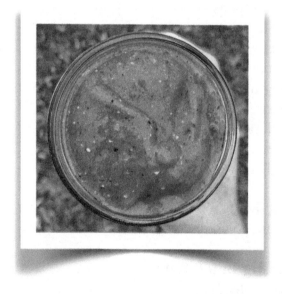

Lunch
<u>Seasonal fruits of choice</u>, for example:
Spring: bowl of 2 chopped apricots & 3 sliced bananas
Summer: bowl of 1/2 of a papaya & 1 sliced banana
Autumn: bowl of grapes, 1 chopped apples, & 2 sliced bananas
Winter: bowl of 4 sliced oranges & 2 chopped apples

Day 8, cont'd.

Dinner
<u>Sweet Masala Salad</u>
1 large head of red leaf lettuce, chopped
1 cup red cabbage, shredded
1/4 cup parsley, chopped
1/4 cup yellow onion, chopped
2 carrots, shredded or chopped
1/2 cucumber, chopped
7 - 10 grape tomatoes, whole or sliced

<u>Sweet Masala Dressing</u>
3 Tbsp sesame seeds
1/3 cup red bell pepper, chopped
2 medjool dates, pitted
1/2 lemon, peeled
1 tsp onion granules
2 tsp Frontier Tandoori Masala seasoning
1/4 tsp black pepper
1 pinch cayenne pepper
3/4 cup purified water

Add all ingredients to a blender and blend until smooth.
Pour over your salad and enjoy!

Suggested Big Batch Side
<u>Spaghetti and Meatless Balls</u>
Enjoy serving #2 of 3 of your leftovers.

If desired, place in a dehydrator set at 105 degrees
Fahrenheit for 1 - 2 hours to soften the noodles and give it a
more traditional pasta mouth-feel.

Day 9

Breakfast
Strawberry Basil Blast
5 - 10 ripe bananas
1 - 2 cups frozen strawberries
1/4 cup basil leaves
1 - 2 tsp chia, flax, or hemp seeds (optional)
1 - 2 cups purified water, or to desired consistency

Add all of the ingredients into your blender.
Blend until smooth.
Enjoy!

Lunch
Seasonal fruits of choice, for
example:
Spring: 2 mangoes & 1/2 of a
pineapple
Summer: 5 mangoes
Autumn: 4 figs & 2 bananas
Winter: 3 apples & 2 bananas

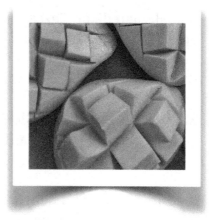

Dinner
Sesame Sour Cream Salad
1/2 large head iceberg lettuce,
chopped
1 - 2 cups arugula, chopped
1/4 cup parsley, chopped
1/4 cup yellow onion, chopped
1/2 to 1 cup frozen green peas, thawed
1/3 cup beet, shredded
2 carrots, shredded or chopped
7 - 10 grape tomatoes, whole or sliced

Day 9, cont'd.

Add all ingredients to a large salad bowl and mix well.

<u>Sesame Sour Cream Dressing</u>
3 Tbsp sesame seeds
2 Medjool dates, pitted
1/2 lemon, peeled
1 tsp garlic granules
1 tsp onion granules
1 tsp dijon mustard
1 Tbsp chives, fresh or dried
 cup purified water

Add all ingredients (except the chives) to a blender and blend until smooth.
Add the chives and pulse until mixed well.
Pour over your salad and enjoy!

Suggested Big Batch Side
<u>Spaghetti and Meatless Balls</u>
Enjoy final serving of your leftovers.

If desired, place in a dehydrator set at 105 degrees Fahrenheit for 1 - 2 hours to soften the noodles and give it a more traditional pasta mouth-feel.

Day 10

Breakfast
Delectable Chocolate Shake
5 - 10 ripe bananas
3 - 4 Medjool dates
2 tsp carob powder
1 - 2 tsp chia, flax, or hemp seeds (optional)
1 - 2 cups purified water, or to desired consistency

Add all of the ingredients into your blender.
Blend until smooth.
Enjoy!

Lunch
Seasonal fruits of choice, for example:
Spring: bowl of 3 sliced bananas & 2 chopped kiwis
Summer: 3 peaches & bowl of blueberries
Autumn: bowl of grapes & 2 apples
Winter: bowl of 3 chopped apples & 3 sliced oranges

Dinner
Sunshine Curry Salad
1/2 large head iceberg lettuce, chopped
1 cup red cabbage, shredded
1/4 cup basil, chopped
1/4 cup yellow onion, chopped
1/2 to 1 cup frozen corn, thawed
1/3 cup beet, shredded
2 stalks celery, chopped
7 - 10 grape tomatoes, whole or sliced

Sunshine Curry Dressing
3 Tbsp sesame seeds
1/2 lemon, peeled

Day 10, cont'd.

3 Medjool dates, pitted
2 tsp curry powder
1 tsp onion granules
1/4 tsp black pepper (or to taste)
1/2 jalapeno, chopped (remove seeds, if desired)
3/4 cup purified water

Add all ingredients to a blender and blend until smooth.
Pour over your salad and enjoy!

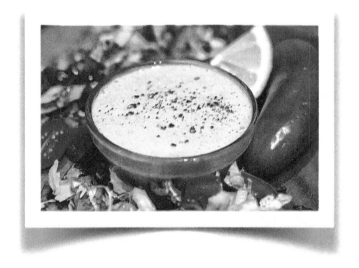

Suggested Big Batch Side
Zettucine Alfredo and Meatless Balls
Makes 3 servings - enjoy 1 serving and save the rest for Days
11 and 12.

Components:
5 large zucchini
1 cup of Hemp Garlic Sauce
3 Tbsp Raw Walnut Meat

Day 10, cont'd.

Making the Zettucine Noodles:
Use a spiralizer or a julienne peeler to turn your 5 zucchini into noodles - peel the skin from the zucchini before spiralizing.
Place your zettucine noodles in a mixing bowl.

Hemp Garlic Sauce:
1/3 cup hemp seeds
1 cup peeled zucchini, chopped
1 clove garlic
1/4 cup yellow onion
3 Tbsp nutritional yeast
1 heaping tsp black pepper
1 tsp organic miso or 1 tsp sea salt
1 tsp psyllium husk powder
1 cup distilled water

Add all ingredients to a blender and blend until smooth.
Add 1 cup of Hemp Garlic Sauce to the mixing bowl.

Raw Walnut Meat:
3/4 cup walnuts, soaked in water for 4 - 8 hours then rinsed
3/4 cup sunflower seeds, soaked in water for 4 - 8 hours then rinsed
3/4 cup sun-dried tomatoes, soaked in water for 1 hour
1 cup sweet onion, chopped
1/2 cup parsley, chopped
2 tsp thyme
2 tsp sage
2 tsp paprika
2 tsp chili powder
1 clove garlic

Day 10, cont'd.

Place all ingredients (except the chopped parsley) into a food processor with the "s-blade" and process until thoroughly combined.
Add the chopped parsley and pulse until it is well combined with the rest of the mixture.
Add 1 - 3 Tbsp of Walnut Meat to the mixing bowl.

Mix well until everything is thoroughly combined.
Serve and enjoy!

If desired, place the final mixture in a dehydrator set at 105 degrees Fahrenheit for 1 - 2 hours to soften the noodles and give it a more traditional pasta mouth-feel. You can also omit the Raw Walnut Meat for a fat free version of this recipe.

Store leftovers in glass containers in the fridge for up to 5 days.

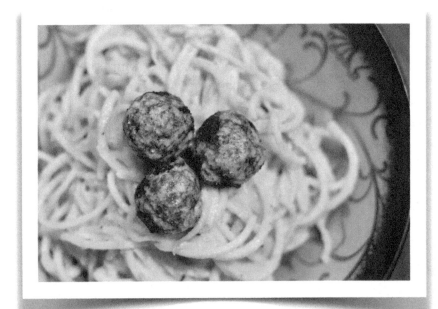

Day 11

Breakfast

Strawberry Mango Splash

5 - 10 ripe bananas

1 cup frozen strawberries

1 cup frozen mango

1 tsp chlorella powder

1 - 2 tsp chia, flax, or hemp seeds (optional)

1 - 2 cups purified water, or to desired consistency

Add all of the ingredients into your blender.

Blend until smooth.

Enjoy!

Lunch

Seasonal fruits of choice, for example:

Spring: 3 mangoes & 1 banana

Summer: bowl of 3 chopped plums & raspberries

Autumn: 2 persimmons & 2 apples

Winter: bowl of 4 sliced bananas & 2 handfuls of dried mulberries

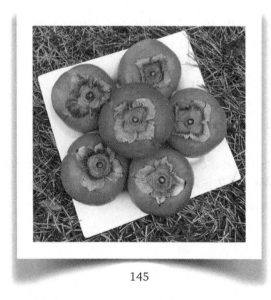

Day 11, cont'd.

Dinner
Chili Brazily Salad
1 large head red leaf lettuce, chopped
1 - 2 cups arugula, chopped
1/4 cup parsley, chopped
1/4 cup yellow onion, chopped
1/2 cucumber, sliced or chopped
1/2 to 1 cup frozen green peas, thawed
1/2 cup button mushrooms, chopped
2 carrots, chopped
7 - 10 grape tomatoes, whole or sliced

Chili Brazily Dressing
3 Tbsp brazil nuts
2 medjool dates, pitted
1/2 lemon, peeled
1 tsp onion granules
1 tsp chili powder
1 tsp yellow mustard
1 cup purified water

Add all ingredients to a blender and blend until smooth.
Pour over your salad and enjoy!

Suggested Big Batch Side
Zettucine Alfredo and Meatless Balls
Enjoy serving #2 of 3 of your leftovers.

If desired, place in a dehydrator set at 105 degrees
Fahrenheit for 1 - 2 hours to soften the noodles and give it a
more traditional pasta mouth-feel.

Day 12

Breakfast

<u>Cherry Berry Bonanza</u>
5 - 10 ripe bananas
1 cup frozen cherries
1 cup frozen strawberries
1 cup arugula
1 - 2 tsp chia, flax, or hemp seeds (optional)
1 - 2 cups purified water, or to desired consistency

Add all of the ingredients into your blender.
Blend until smooth.
Enjoy!

Lunch

<u>Seasonal fruits of choice</u>, for example:
Spring: bowl of 3
sliced bananas,
blueberries, &
raspberries
Summer: 4 mangoes &
a few cherries
Autumn: bowl of 2
peeled pomegranates
& 3 chopped apples
Winter: bowl of 3
chopped pears & 2
sliced bananas

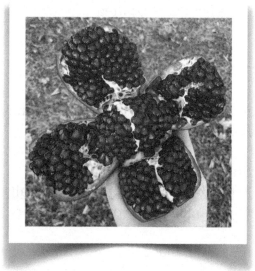

Day 12, cont'd.

Dinner:
<u>Chipotle Almond Salad</u>
1/2 large head iceberg lettuce, chopped
1 cup red cabbage, shredded
1/4 cup basil, chopped
1/4 cup yellow onion, chopped
1/2 cucumber, chopped
1/2 - 1 cup frozen corn, thawed
2 carrots, shredded or chopped
7 - 10 grape tomatoes, whole or sliced

Add all ingredients to a large salad bowl and mix well.

<u>Chipotle Almond Dressing</u>
3 Tbsp almonds
1/2 lemon, peeled
2 Medjool dates, pitted
1/2 tsp chipotle powder
1 tsp dijon mustard
3/4 cup purified water

Add all ingredients to a blender and blend until smooth.
Pour over your salad and enjoy!

Suggested Big Batch Side
<u>Zettucine Alfredo and Meatless Balls</u>
Enjoy final serving of your leftovers.

If desired, place in a dehydrator set at 105 degrees
Fahrenheit for 1 - 2 hours to soften the noodles and give it a
more traditional pasta mouth-feel.

Day 13

Breakfast
<u>Tropical Celebration</u>
5 - 10 ripe bananas
1 - 2 cups frozen mango
2 - 3 Medjool dates
2 stalks celery
1 - 2 tsp chia, flax, or hemp seeds (optional)
1 - 2 cups purified water, or to desired consistency

Add all of the ingredients into your blender.
Blend until smooth.
Enjoy!

Lunch
<u>Seasonal fruits of choice</u>, for example:
Spring: 2 apricots & 1/2 of a pineapple
Summer: bowl of 1/2 of a
chopped papaya & 1 sliced
banana
Autumn: 3 apples & 4 figs
Winter: 4 pears

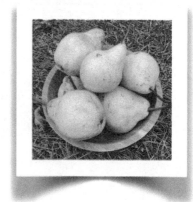

Dinner
<u>Sagemary Salad</u>
1/2 large head iceberg lettuce,
chopped
1 - 2 cups arugula, chopped
1/4 cup parsley, chopped
1/4 cup yellow onion, chopped
1/3 beet, shredded
1/2 cucumber, chopped
2 carrots, shredded or chopped
7 - 10 grape tomatoes, whole or sliced

Day 13, cont'd.

<u>Sagemary Dressing</u>
3 Tbsp sunflower seeds
1/2 lemon, peeled
2 Medjool dates, pitted
1 clove garlic
1 tsp onion granules
1 tsp dried rosemary
1 tsp dried sage
Pinch of cayenne pepper (to taste)
3/4 cup purified water

Add all ingredients to a blender and blend until smooth.
Pour over your salad and enjoy!

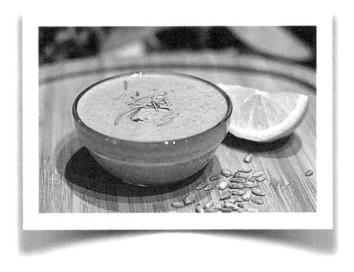

Suggested Big Batch Side
<u>Angeled Tomatoes</u>
Makes 4 servings - enjoy 4 to 5 halved angeled tomatoes and
save the rest for Days 14 and 15.

Day 13, cont'd.

1 cups cashews, soaked in water for 4 - 8 hours then rinsed
2 Tbsp yellow mustard
1 Medjool date, pitted
1 tsp smoked paprika
1 tsp onion powder
2 tsp dried dill
1/2 tsp turmeric powder
1 tsp black pepper
1/2 tsp sea salt
2 Tbsp apple cider vinegar
1/2 cup water
10 small Roma tomatoes

Add all ingredients (except tomatoes) to a blender and blend until smooth.
Slice each tomato in half (length-wise) and scoop out the middle with a spoon - add this to your salad!
With a spoon, add the blended mixture into the center of each slice of tomato and top with an additional pinch of smoked paprika.
Serve and enjoy.

Store leftovers in a glass container in the fridge for up to 5 days.

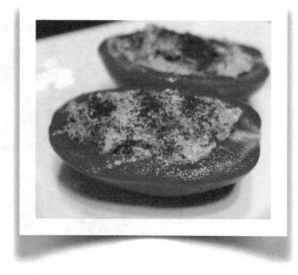

Day 14

Breakfast
<u>Strawberry Shortcake</u>
5 - 10 ripe bananas
1 - 2 cups strawberries
2 - 3 Medjool dates
2 tsp maca powder
1 - 2 tsp chia, flax, or hemp seeds (optional)
1 - 2 cups purified water, or to desired consistency

Add all of the ingredients into your blender.
Blend until smooth.
Enjoy!

Lunch
<u>Seasonal fruits of choice</u>, for example:
Spring: 2 mangoes & 1/2 of a pineapple
Summer: 1 watermelon
Autumn: 1 papaya
Winter: 5 dates & 2 bananas

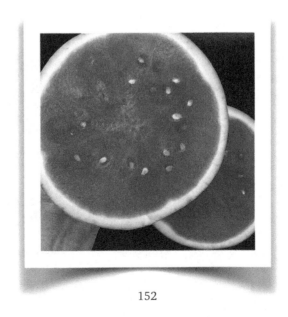

Day 14, cont'd.

Dinner

<u>Brazilian Maca Salad</u>
1 large head red leaf lettuce, chopped
1 cup red cabbage, shredded
1/4 cup parsley, chopped
1 cup frozen organic corn, thawed
1/4 cup yellow onion, chopped
½ jalapeño, chopped (remove seeds, if desired)
2 carrots, chopped
7 - 10 grape tomatoes, whole or sliced

Add all ingredients to a large salad bowl and mix well.

<u>Brazilian Maca Dressing</u>
3 Tbsp Brazil nuts
1/2 lemon, peeled
2 Medjool dates, pitted
1 clove garlic
1 tsp maca
1 tsp onion granules
1 cup purified water

Add all ingredients to a blender and blend until smooth.
Pour over your salad and enjoy!

Suggested Big Batch Side
<u>Angeled Tomatoes</u>
Enjoy serving #2 of 3 of your leftovers.

Day 15

Breakfast
<u>Hawaiian Green</u>
5 - 10 ripe bananas
1 cup frozen pineapple
1 cup frozen mango
1 cup spinach
1 - 2 tsp chia, flax, or hemp seeds (optional)
1 - 2 cups purified water, or to desired consistency

Add all of the ingredients into your blender.
Blend until smooth.
Enjoy!

Lunch
<u>Seasonal fruits of choice</u>, for example:
Spring: bowl of 2 sliced mango & 1/2 of a pineapple
Summer: 3 peaches & bowl of blueberries
Autumn: 2 pomegranates & large bowl of grapes
Winter: 3 apples & 1 pear

Dinner
<u>Rawnch Salad</u>
1 large head romaine lettuce, chopped
1 - 2 cups bok choy, chopped
1/4 cup dill, chopped
1/4 cup red onion, chopped
2 stalks celery, chopped
1/2 to 1 cup frozen green peas, thawed
2 carrots, shredded or chopped
7 - 10 grape tomatoes, whole or sliced

Add all ingredients to a large salad bowl and mix well.

Day 15, cont'd.

Rawnch Dressing
3 Tbsp hemp seeds
1 medium zucchini, peeled
1 tsp garlic granules
1 tsp onion granules
1 tsp dried dill
1 tsp chickpea miso
2 tsp chives, fresh or dried
1/2 lemon, peeled
1 tsp black pepper
1 tsp psyllium husk powder
3/4 cup purified water

Add all ingredients in a blender and blend until smooth.
Pour on your salad and enjoy!
Suggested Big Batch Side
Angeled Tomatoes
Enjoy final serving of your leftovers.

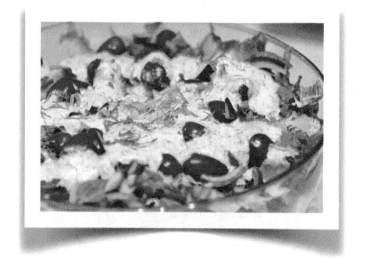

Day 16

Breakfast:

<u>Blueberry Kale Infusion</u>
5 - 10 ripe bananas
1 - 2 cups frozen blueberries
2 - 3 Medjool dates
1 cup kale
1 - 2 tsp chia, flax, or hemp seeds (optional)
1 - 2 cups purified water, or to desired consistency

Add all of the ingredients into your blender.
Blend until smooth.
Enjoy!

Lunch

<u>Seasonal fruits of choice</u>, for example:
Spring: bowl of 3 chopped peaches & blueberries
Summer: 5 plums & bowl of cherries
Autumn: 4 persimmons & 2 apples
Winter: 5 oranges & 1 apple

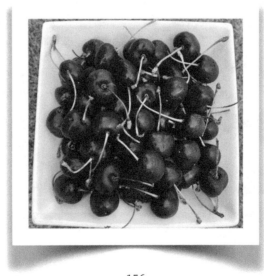

Day 16, cont'd.

Dinner

<u>Avocado, Corn, and Herb Salad</u>
10 oz spinach, chopped
1 - 2 cups kale, finely chopped
1/4 cup cilantro, chopped
1/4 cup red onion, chopped
1/2 cucumber, chopped
1/2 to 1 cup frozen organic corn, thawed
2 carrots, shredded or chopped
7 - 10 grape tomatoes, whole or sliced

Add all ingredients to a large salad bowl and mix well.

<u>Avocado Herb Dressing</u>
1 medium hass avocado, mashed
1/2 lemon, juice only
2 tsp yellow mustard
1 Tbsp Kirkland's Organic No Salt Seasoning
Red pepper chili flakes to taste (optional)

Mix together until well combined.
Mix into your salad and enjoy!

Suggested Big Batch Side

<u>Veggie Loaf</u>
Makes 3 servings - enjoy 1 serving and save the rest for Days 17 and 18.

Loaf:
4 medium carrots, chopped
3 large stalks celery, chopped
2 cups frozen green peas, thawed
8 medium button mushrooms, chopped

Day 16, cont'd.

1 cup sun-dried tomatoes, soaked in water for 20 minutes
then drained
1 cup sweet onion, chopped
2 garlic cloves, pressed or finely chopped
1/2 cup walnuts, soaked in water for 4 - 8 hours then rinsed
2 tsp paprika
2 tsp cumin
2 Tbsp chia seeds, ground
1 batch of Raw Ketchup

Raw Ketchup:
1 ½ cups grape tomatoes or 5 Roma tomatoes
1/2 cup sun-dried tomatoes, soaked in water for 1 hour
3 Medjool dates, pitted
2 tsp onion granules
2 Tbsp apple cider vinegar

Add all ingredients to a blender and blend until smooth.
Set Raw Ketchup to the side for now.

Add 2 Tbsp chia seeds to a high-speed blender or coffee
grinder and grind into powder.
Add all ingredients (except ketchup) to a food processor and
process until mixed well.
Place the processed mixture onto a dehydrator tray with a
teflex sheet and split into 3 equal parts.
Form the 3 portions of mixture into about 1-inch thick loaves.
Dehydrate at 105 degrees for 3 hours.
After 3 hours, remove the tray from the dehydrator and place
another dehydrator tray without the teflex sheet on top of
your 3 loaves, essentially sandwiching the loaves

Day 16, cont'd.

between the two dehydrator trays. Now, quickly but carefully flip the two trays over and remove the top tray along with the teflex sheet. The loaves will now be bottom up.

Place the tray with the loaves back into the dehydrator for 2 ½ hours.

Remove the tray from the dehydrator and apply a thin layer of ketchup on top of each loaf.

Place back into the dehydrator for 30 minutes.

Remove the loaves from the dehydrator, serve, and enjoy.

Store leftovers in a glass container in the fridge for up to 5 days.

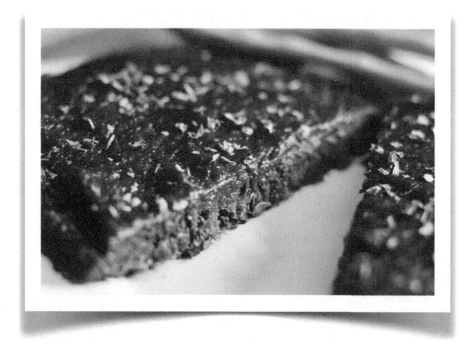

Day 17

Breakfast
Pineapple Berry Awakening
5 - 10 ripe bananas
1 cup frozen pineapple
1 cup frozen strawberries
1 - 2 tsp chia, flax, or hemp seeds (optional)
1 - 2 cups purified water, or to desired consistency

Add all of the ingredients into your blender.
Blend until smooth.
Enjoy!

Lunch
Seasonal fruits of choice, for example:
Spring: bowl of 2 sliced mangoes & 2 sliced bananas
Summer: 1 honeydew or cantaloupe melon
Autumn: 1 papaya
Winter: 4 apples, handful of dates, & celery sticks

Dinner
Brazilian Curry Salad
1 large head green leaf lettuce, chopped
1 - 2 cups bok choy, chopped
1/4 cup dill, chopped
1/4 cup red onion, chopped
2 carrots, shredded or chopped
1/2 to 1 cup frozen peas, thawed
1/2 cucumber, chopped
7 - 10 grape tomatoes, whole or sliced

Add all ingredients to a large salad bowl and mix well.

Day 17, cont'd.

<u>Brazilian Curry Dressing</u>
3 Tbsp Brazil nuts
1 cloves garlic
2 Medjool dates, pitted
1/2 lemon, peeled
1 tsp curry powder
Pinch of cinnamon
1 tsp yellow mustard
1 cup purified water

Add all ingredients to a blender and blend until smooth.
Pour over your salad and enjoy!

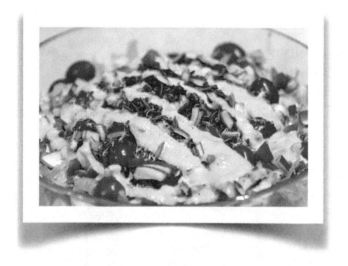

Suggested Big Batch Side
<u>Veggie Loaf</u>
Enjoy serving #2 of 3 of your leftovers.

Warm in the dehydrator at 105 degrees Fahrenheit for up to a
couple of hours to give it a slightly warmer feel.

Day 18

Breakfast

Sweet Detox

5 - 10 ripe bananas
1 - 2 cups frozen blueberries
2 - 3 Medjool dates
1/4 cup cilantro
1 tsp chlorella
1 - 2 tsp chia, flax, or hemp seeds (optional)
1 - 2 cups purified water, or to desired consistency

Add all of the ingredients into your blender.
Blend until smooth.
Enjoy!

Lunch

Seasonal fruits of choice, for example:
Spring: 3 kiwis & 1/2 of a pineapple
Summer: bowl of 1/2 of a papaya & 1 sliced banana
Autumn: bowl of 3 sliced persimmons & 2 sliced bananas
Winter: bowl of 3 sliced bananas, handful of dried mulberries, & cinnamon

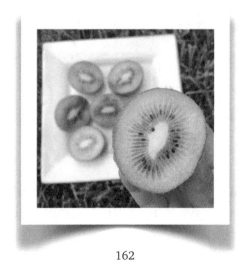

Day 18, cont'd.

Dinner:
<u>Cajun Red Salad</u>
1 large head green leaf lettuce, chopped
1 - 2 cups kale, chopped
1/4 cup cilantro, chopped
1/4 cup red onion, chopped
1/2 cucumber, chopped
2 carrots, chopped
7 - 10 grape tomatoes, whole or sliced

Add all ingredients to a large salad bowl and mix well.

<u>Cajun Red Dressing</u>
3 Tbsp almonds
2 Medjool dates, pitted
1/2 lemon, peeled
1 tsp onion granules
1 tsp paprika
2 tsp Dijon mustard
1/2 tsp Cajun seasoning
3/4 cup water

Add all ingredients to a blender and blend until smooth,
Pour over your salad and enjoy!

Suggested Big Batch Side
<u>Veggie Loaf</u>
Enjoy final serving of your leftovers.

Warm in the dehydrator at 105 degrees Fahrenheit for up to a
couple of hours to give it a slightly warmer feel.

Day 19

Breakfast
<u>Carob Berry Pie</u>
5 - 10 ripe bananas
1 - 2 cups frozen strawberries
2 - 3 Medjool dates
1 Tbsp carob powder
1 - 2 tsp chia, flax, or hemp seeds (optional)
1 - 2 cups purified water, or to desired consistency

Add all of the ingredients into your blender.
Blend until smooth.
Enjoy!

Lunch
<u>Seasonal fruits of choice</u>, for example:
Spring: bowl of 3 sliced apricots & 2 sliced mangoes
Summer: 5 mangoes
Autumn: 2 apples & 5 figs
Winter: 6 oranges & dried mango slices

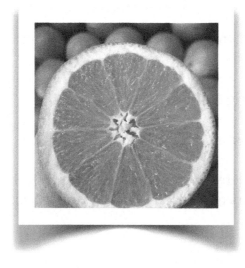

Day 19, cont'd.

Dinner
Royal Dragon Salad
1 large head romaine lettuce, chopped
1 - 2 cups bok choy, chopped
1/4 cup cilantro, chopped
1/4 cup red onion, chopped
1/3 cup celery, chopped
1/2 to 1 cup frozen peas, thawed
1/3 cup button mushrooms, chopped or sliced
2 carrots, shredded or chopped
7 - 10 grape tomatoes, whole or sliced

Add all ingredients to a large salad bowl and mix well.

Royal Dragon Dressing
3 Tbsp sesame seeds
1/2 lemon, peeled
2 Medjool dates, pitted
2 tsp Dijon mustard
1/2 inch fresh ginger
1 clove garlic
1 tsp paprika
1/4 tsp cayenne pepper (or to taste)
3/4 cup water

Add all ingredients to a blender and blend until smooth.
Pour over your salad and enjoy!

Suggested Big Batch Side
Wild Rice Stuffing
Makes 3 large servings - enjoy 1 serving (this equals a volume
of around 2 bowls) and save the rest for Days 20 and 21.

Day 19, cont'd.

2 cups bloomed wild rice
1/2 cup soaked almonds
2 carrots
2 stalks celery
1/3 cup sweet onion
1 Tbsp lemon juice
2 tsp dried sage
2 tsp dried oregano
2 tsp dried thyme
1/4 cup fresh parsley, chopped
1 tsp apple cider vinegar or an additional 1 Tbsp lemon juice
1/4 cup water

Soak at least one cup of wild rice in 4 cups of clean water for 24 to 36 hours. This will give you about 2 cups of bloomed wild rice.
**To help your wild rice bloom better, you can run it through the food processor with the "S-blade" for about 1 minute before soaking. This puts small cuts in the outer layer of the rice and allows water to get inside easier to help it bloom.
Test the wild rice to make sure it has become soft and chewy. Many of the seeds should have broken open, showing the white inner portion.
When ready, drain the wild rice well and add two cups into a large mixing bowl and set to the side.
Place the almonds in a food processor and process with the S-blade until finely chopped.
Add the chopped almonds to your mixing bowl.
One at a time, in the food processor with the S-blade, finely chop the carrots, celery, onions, and parsley.

Day 19, cont'd.

Add everything to the mixing bowl as you finish chopping each ingredient.

With a knife or in the food processor, finely chop the fresh parsley and add into the mixing bowl.

Add the sage, oregano, thyme, apple cider vinegar (or lemon juice), and water to the mixing bowl.

Mix everything very well.

Serve and enjoy.

Store leftovers in a glass container in the fridge for up to 5 days.

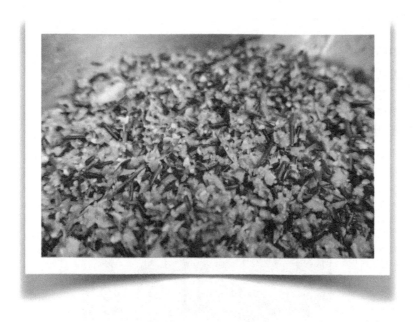

Day 20

Breakfast
Divine Sunrise
5 - 10 ripe bananas
1 cup frozen pineapple
1 - 2 navel oranges
1 cup spinach
1 - 2 tsp chia, flax, or hemp seeds (optional)
1 - 2 cups purified water, or to desired consistency

Add all of the ingredients into your blender.
Blend until smooth.
Enjoy!

Lunch
Seasonal fruits of choice, for example:
Spring: 3 apricots & 2 bananas
Summer: 3 nectarines & a bowl of strawberries
Autumn: 2 pomegranates & 1 apple
Winter: 3 pears & 2 apples

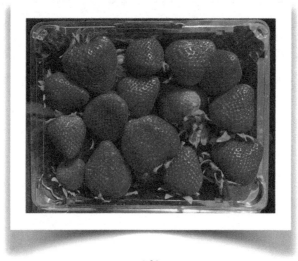

Day 20, cont'd.

Dinner

Buttermylk Salad

1 large head romaine lettuce, chopped
1 - 2 cups kale, finely chopped
1/4 cup dill, chopped
1/4 cup red onion, chopped
2 stalks celery, chopped
2 carrots, shredded or chopped
7 - 10 grape tomatoes, whole or sliced

Add all ingredients to a large salad bowl and mix well.

Buttermylk Dressing

3 Tbsp sesame seeds
3 medjool dates, pitted
1/2 lemon, peeled
1 Tbsp brown mustard
3/4 cup water

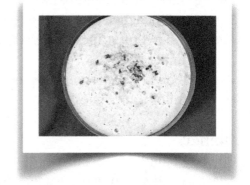

Add all ingredients to a
blender and blend until
smooth.
Pour over your salad and
enjoy!

**Suggested Big Batch
Side**

Wild Rice Stuffing
Enjoy serving #2 of 3 of your leftovers.

Day 21

Breakfast
<u>Solar Burst</u>
5 - 10 ripe bananas
1 - 2 cups frozen mango
1 - 2 navel oranges
1 - 2 cups kale
1 - 2 tsp chia, flax, or hemp seeds (optional)
1 - 2 cups purified water, or to desired consistency

Add all of the ingredients into your blender.
Blend until smooth.
Enjoy!

Lunch
<u>Seasonal fruits of choice</u>, for example:
Spring: bowl of 3 sliced bananas, strawberries, & blueberries
Summer: 3 peaches & a bowl of blueberries
Autumn: bowl of grapes, 2 sliced pears, & seeds of 1 pomegranate
Winter: bowl of 2 chopped apples, 1 chopped pear, 1 banana, & handful of mulberries

Dinner:
<u>Cowboy Salad</u>
1 large head green leaf lettuce, chopped
1 - 2 cups bok choy, chopped
1/4 cup cilantro, chopped
1/4 cup red onion, chopped
1/2 to 1 cup frozen green peas, thawed
1/2 cucumber, chopped
2 carrots, chopped
7 - 10 grape tomatoes, whole or sliced

Day 21, cont'd.

Add all ingredients to a large salad bowl and mix well.

Cowboy Sauce
3 Tbsp sesame seeds
1/3 cup red bell pepper
2 Medjool dates, pitted
1 clove garlic
1/2 lemon, peeled
1 tsp paprika
1/2 tsp red pepper flakes
3/4 cup water

Add all ingredients to a blender and blend until smooth.
Pour over your salad and enjoy!

Suggested Big Batch Side
Wild Rice Stuffing
Enjoy final serving of your leftovers.

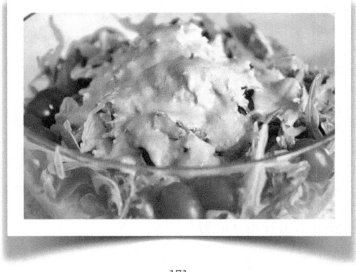

Recipes

Snacks

Banana Cinnamon Rolls
Caramel Date Sauce:
15 Medjool dates, pitted
1/4 tsp cinnamon
1/2 cup purified water

Add all ingredients to a blender and blend until smooth.

Cinnamon Rolls:
5 - 6 ripe bananas

Cut the bananas lengthwise into three slices.
Lay flat on a dehydrator tray with a teflex sheet and dehydrate at 105 degrees Fahrenheit for 6 hours - or until they are flexible enough to bend without breaking.
Spread caramel date sauce along each strip of dried banana and roll them up.
Place back in the dehydrator for 2 - 4 hours and enjoy!
Store leftovers in a glass container in the fridge for up to 5 days.

Blueberry Nice Cream
4 frozen bananas
1 cup frozen blueberries
Additional fresh blueberries for topping (optional)

Add frozen bananas and frozen blueberries to a food processor and process until it resembles soft-serve ice cream.
Top with fresh blueberries
Serve immediately and enjoy.

Chocolate Mulberry Crunch Balls
15 Medjool dates (pitted)
3/4 cup dried mulberries
1 Tbsp carob powder

Add all ingredients to a food processor and process until thoroughly combined.
Form the mixture into many small balls - should make about 20 - 25 small balls.
Tip: Dip your fingers in a bowl of purified water before rolling each ball to prevent the mixture from getting too sticky.
Serve and enjoy!
Store the leftovers in a glass container in the freezer for up to several weeks.

Caramel Apples
2 - 3 apples of choice, sliced
15 Medjool dates pitted
1/4 tsp cinnamon (optional)
1/2 cup purified water

Add the dates, cinnamon, and water to a blender and blend until smooth to make Caramel Date Sauce.
Slice the apples and dip into the date sauce.
Enjoy!
Store leftovers in a glass container in the fridge for up to 5 days.

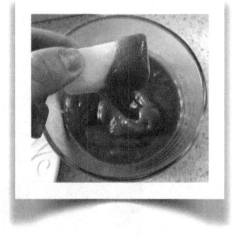

Fresh Sprouts

Homegrown sprouts make a great snack. My favorites are green peas and french lentil sprouts.

Soak 1/3 cup of green pea or lentil sprouts in a quart mason jar for 8 hours at room temperature.

Drain the soak water and rinse the seeds.

Place the jar with the mouth angled down at about a 45-degree angle to allow excess water to drain out. You can find lids made specifically for sprouting online or you can use cheese cloth.

For the next 3 - 5 days, while keeping the jars at room temperature, rinse and drain the seeds each morning and night.

They are ready to eat after 3 - 5 days.

Eat as many as desired.

Store leftovers in a glass container in the fridge for 5 to 7 days.

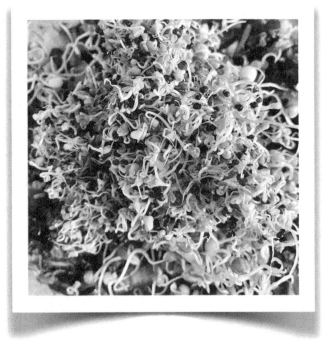

Big Batch Sides

Angeled Tomatoes
Makes 4 servings

1 cup cashews, soaked in water for 4 - 8 hours then rinsed
2 Tbsp yellow mustard
1 Medjool date, pitted
1 tsp smoked paprika
1 tsp onion powder
2 tsp dried dill
1/2 tsp turmeric powder
1 tsp black pepper
1/2 tsp sea salt
2 Tbsp apple cider vinegar
1/2 cup water
10 small Roma tomatoes

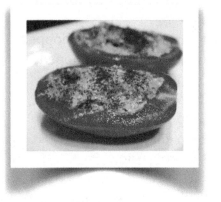

Add all ingredients (except tomatoes) to a blender and blend until smooth.
Slice each tomato in half (length-wise) and scoop out the middle with a spoon - add this to your salad!
With a spoon, add the blended mixture into the center of each slice of tomato and top with an additional pinch of smoked paprika.
Serve and enjoy.

Store leftovers in a glass container in the fridge for up to 5 days.

BBQ Meatless Balls
Makes 10 servings, with 3 balls equaling 1 serving

Meatless balls:
3/4 cup walnuts, soaked in water for 4 - 8 hours then rinsed)
3/4 cup sunflower seeds, soaked in water for 4 - 8 hours, then rinsed)
3/4 cup sun-dried tomatoes, soaked in water for at least 1 hour
1 cup sweet onion, chopped
1/2 cup parsley, chopped
2 tsp thyme
2 tsp sage
2 tsp paprika
2 tsp chili powder
1 clove garlic

Place all ingredients (except the chopped parsley) into a food processor with the "s-blade" and process until thoroughly combined.
Add the chopped parsley and pulse until it is well combined with the rest of the mixture.
Using a tablespoon, scoop out about 3/4 of a tablespoon of the mixture and form into a ball. This will make roughly 30 balls of this size.
Place the meatless balls evenly spaced apart on a dehydrator tray.

BBQ Sauce:
5 Roma tomatoes
1 cup sun-dried tomatoes, soaked in water for 1 hour
1 clove garlic
3/4 cup sweet onion
5 Medjool dates
1/2 lemon, peeled

2 tsp mustard powder or yellow mustard
2 tsp smoked paprika
1 Tbsp apple cider vinegar

Add all ingredients to a blender and blend until smooth. Using a spoon, scoop out a small amount of BBQ sauce and cover the top of each meatless ball with a thin layer of sauce. Place the tray of BBQ meatless balls into the dehydrator at 105 degrees Fahrenheit for 12 hours.

Add the BBQ meatless balls to pasta, salads, or wraps.

Broccoli Slaw
4 cups small broccoli florets
3 cups red cabbage, chopped
2 carrots, shredded
1 cup raisins (oil free)
1/2 cup walnuts, soaked for 8 hours in water then rinsed
1/3 cup maple syrup
1/4 cup apple cider vinegar (optional)
1 lemon, juiced

Chop the broccoli into small bite-sized pieces and place into a large mixing bowl.
In a food processor, pulse the cabbage into small pieces using the "S blade" and place into the mixing bowl.
Shred the carrots and add them to the mixing bowl.
Add the raisins to the mixing bowl.
In the food processor, pulse the walnuts into small pieces and add to the mixing bowl.
In a separate bowl, whisk together the maple syrup, apple cider vinegar, lemon juice and add to the mixing bowl.
Mix well, serve, and enjoy.
Store leftovers in a glass container in the fridge for up to 5 days.

Creamy Broccoli Salad

Dressing:
1 cup cashews
4 Medjool dates
1 lemon, peeled
1 clove garlic
1/2 tsp sea salt
1/2 cup purified water

Place all ingredients in a blender and blend until smooth.

Salad:
4 cups small broccoli florets
2 cups red grapes, sliced into halves
3 stalks celery, chopped
½ cup red onion, chopped
1 cup dried cranberries or raisins (dried, no oil)

Combine all salad ingredients in a large mixing bowl.
Pour the dressing over the salad ingredients and mix thoroughly.
Serve as a side dish to your salad and enjoy!
Store the leftovers in a glass container in the fridge for up to 5 days.

Cucumber Dill Rollups

1 avocado, mashed
2 green onions, finely chopped
1 red bell pepper, sliced
1 Tbsp lemon juice
2 Tbsp fresh dill, finely chopped
2 cucumbers
Optional: using a julienne peeler, slice the outside layer of the red bell pepper into strips and place to the side for later.

Add the remaining red bell pepper, green onion, dill, and lemon juice to the food processor and pulse until finely chopped.

Add the avocado to the food processor and pulse again until everything is mixed, and it resembles guacamole.

Using a vegetable peeler, slice the cucumbers lengthwise into long, thin strips.

Add a thin layer of the avocado mixture to each cucumber strip.

Add a few of the thin red bell pepper strips to the left edge of the cucumber slices (so the pepper strips hang over the edge).

Starting at the left, gently roll up the strips, being careful not to squeeze out the cucumber filling.

Serve and enjoy.

Store any leftovers in an airtight container in the fridge for up to 36 hours.

Cucumber Mango Pasta

2 large cucumbers, peeled and noodled
2 ataulfo mangoes, skin removed & sliced
*2 cups of frozen mango can be thawed and used if you don't have ataulfo mangoes.
1 cup tomatoes, chopped
1 medium to large avocado, mashed
1 lime or lemon, juiced
1/4 cup cilantro, chopped
1 jalapeño, seeds removed and chopped

With a spiralizer or julienne peeler, turn your peeled cucumber into noodles and place in a bowl.

Cut around the seed of your mango, leaving two "cheeks" of mango. With a knife, gently slice thin strips, without cutting through the skin of the mango. With a spoon, scoop out the strips of mango down to the skin and place into your bowl.

Add your chopped tomatoes and chopped jalapeño to the bowl.
Combine your avocado, cilantro, and lime (or lemon) juice, and mash into guacamole, then add to your bowl.
Combine everything well and enjoy!
Store leftovers in an air-tight, glass container in the fridge for up to 24 hours.

Fen-Apple Slaw
1/2 head of a small red cabbage, finely chopped
2 large apples (any sweet variety)
1 medium bulb fresh fennel, finely chopped
1/2 cup cilantro, finely chopped
1 cup cranberries, fresh or dried
2 Tbsp lemon juice

Finely chop the cabbage in a food processor and place into a mixing bowl.
Repeat above step with the apples.
Repeat above step with the fennel.
Repeat above step with the cilantro, or chop by hand.
Add the lemon juice and cranberries to the mixture, thoroughly mix all ingredients and serve.
Raisins can be substituted for the cranberries if desired.
Store the leftovers in a glass container in the fridge for up to 5 days.

Nori Rocket Wraps and Spicy Thai Almond Sauce
2 - 3 cups arugula
1 avocado, mashed
2 - 3 Tbsp Kim Chi or Sauerkraut
1 cup tomatoes, chopped
3 carrots, shredded
2 - 4 nori wraps

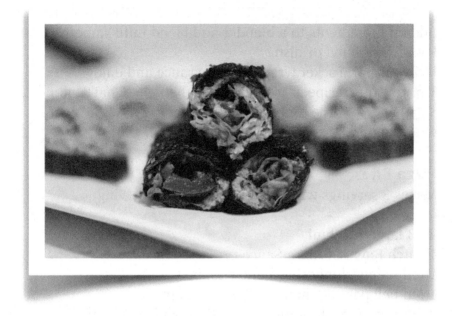

Rough chop the arugula and add to a mixing bowl.
Add the kimchi (or sauerkraut), chopped tomatoes, shredded carrot, and mashed avocado to the mixing bowl and combine everything thoroughly.
Divide the mixture between 2 - 4 nori sheets and roll them up like sushi.
Cut each nori wrap into several sections.

Spicy Thai Almond Sauce:
3 Tbsp almonds, soaked in water for roughly 8 hours then rinsed
1/2 lemon, peeled
1/4 to 1/2 inch fresh ginger, skin removed
2 Medjool dates, pitted
1 tsp red pepper flakes
1 tsp garlic granules
1 tsp organic miso
1/4 tsp paprika
3/4 cup purified water

Add all ingredients to a blender and blend until smooth.
Pour into a bowl or dish.
Dip your nori rocket wraps into the sauce and enjoy!
Tip: Use this recipe as a side dish to the <u>Spicy Thai Almond Salad</u> and split the dipping sauce, using half to dip your wraps and half as the dressing to the salad.

Pizza Bites
Makes 3 servings with 6 - 7 pizza bites per serving

2 - 3 large zucchini
1 batch Raw Marinara Sauce
1 red onion, thinly sliced and chopped
1 red bell pepper, thinly sliced and chopped
2 - 3 button mushrooms, thinly sliced and chopped
Nutritional yeast (optional)
A pinch of red pepper chili flakes (sprinkled on each pizza bite)

Raw Marinara Sauce:
1 ½ cups grape tomatoes or 5 Roma tomatoes
1/2 cup sun-dried tomatoes, soaked in water for 1 hour
3 Medjool dates, pitted
2 tsp onion granules
2 Tbsp apple cider vinegar
2 Tbsp Frontier Pizza Seasoning

Add all ingredients to a blender and blend until smooth.
Using a vegetable peeler, slice your zucchini lengthwise into strips.
Spread a thin layer of raw marinara sauce along the top of each zucchini strip.
Sprinkle with your desired amount of red pepper chili flakes onto the sauce.

Add sliced pieces of red onion, red bell pepper, and mushroom evenly over the marinara.

From the end closest to you, gently but firmly, roll the zucchini slice all the way down the strip.

Be careful not to push or squeeze out the filling ingredients as you roll it.

Place each finished pizza bite on a dehydrator tray with the mesh liner.

Dehydrate at 105 degrees Fahrenheit for 4 hours.

Remove from the dehydrator and enjoy!

Store leftovers in the fridge for 3 - 5 days.

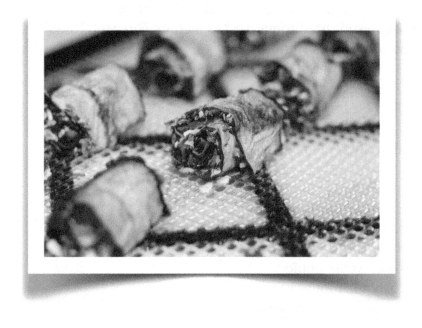

Raw Vegan Lasagna
Makes roughly 3 - 4 servings

This recipe is made best with a special tool called the Vasta or any other vegetable sheet cutting tool:
https://www.amazon.com/s?
k=vasta&crid=261EMRHLEQB70&sprefix=vasta%2Caps%2
C99&ref=nb_sb_noss_2

You can also use a regular veggie peeler and overlap several slices to make the "pasta veggie sheets."

Raw Marinara Sauce:
1 ½ cups grape tomatoes or 5 Roma tomatoes
1/2 cup sun-dried tomatoes (soaked in water for 1 hour)
3 Medjool dates (pitted)
2 tsp onion granules
2 Tbsp apple cider vinegar
2 Tbsp Frontier Pizza Seasoning

Add all ingredients to a blender and blend until smooth.

Hemp Garlic Sauce:
1/3 cup hemp seeds
1 cup peeled zucchini, chopped
1 clove garlic
1/4 cup yellow onion
3 Tbsp nutritional yeast
1 heaping tsp black pepper
1 tsp organic miso or 1 tsp sea salt
1 tsp psyllium husk powder
1 cup distilled water

Add all ingredients to a blender and blend until smooth.

Filling Ingredients:
4 button mushrooms
4 Roma tomatoes
2 cups spinach

Veggie Sheets:
2 - 4 zucchini
You will need 3 square sheets for each piece of lasagna.
Start by placing one veggie sheet down and covering with a thin layer of marinara sauce.
Place thin slices of mushroom down so they cover the whole area of the veggie sheet.
Place thin slices of Roma tomato on top of the mushrooms, covering the whole area.
Spread a thin but generous layer of the hemp garlic sauce over the tomatoes.
Place the second veggie sheet on top of the sauce-covered tomatoes.
Repeat the same layering process that you used for the first section.
Place the third veggie sheet on top and cover with a thin, but generous layer of hemp garlic sauce.
You can either enjoy it now, or you can place it in a dehydrator at 105 degrees Fahrenheit for 1-4 hours.

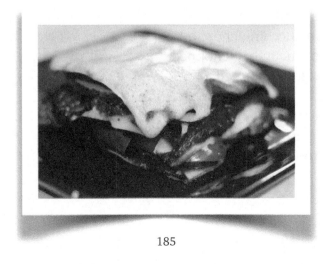

Raw Vegan Vegetable Chili
Makes 3 large servings

Base ingredients:
7 Roma tomatoes
1 cup sun-dried tomatoes, soaked in water for at least 1 hour
1 cup of the soak water
1/2 cup walnuts, soaked in water for 4 - 8 hours then rinsed
1 stalk celery
1 clove garlic
1/3 cup yellow onion
1/2 jalapeño (remove the seeds, if desired)
2 Medjool dates, pitted
1 medium red bell pepper
2 Tbsp thyme
2 Tbsp sweet basil
1 Tbsp chili powder
1 Tbsp cumin

Add all of the base ingredients together in a blender, placing the most water-rich ingredients in the blender first (closest to the blade) and blend until smooth.
Pour into a large mixing bowl and set aside until the chunky ingredients are ready.

Chunky ingredients:
2 medium zucchini, chopped
1 medium cucumber, chopped
4 stalks celery, chopped
3 medium carrots, shredded
5 Roma tomatoes, chopped
1 cup sweet peas
1 cup corn (optional)

Use a food processor to chop (with the S-blade) the zucchini, cucumber, celery, and tomatoes, separately.
Add your chopped ingredients to the mixing bowl that the base mixture is in and mix well.
Use the shredding blade to shred the carrots.
Add the shredded carrots to the mixing bowl.
Add the sweet peas and corn (optional) to the mixing bowl.
Mix everything together very well.
Serve and enjoy.

If desired, place the final mixture in a dehydrator set at 118 degrees Fahrenheit for up to a couple of hours to give it a slightly warmer feel.

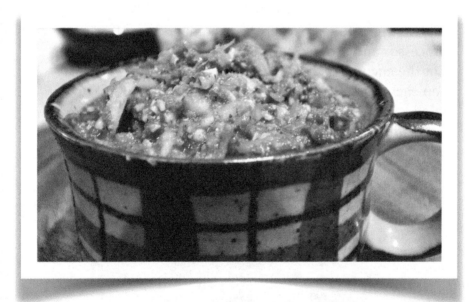

Tuno Sliders
Makes 4 servings

1 - 2 cucumbers
2 large carrots
3 stalks celery
1/2 cup sunflower seeds, soaked for 4 - 8 hours then rinsed
1/2 cup almonds, soaked for 8 hours then rinsed
1/2 cup yellow onion, chopped
Juice of 1 lemon
1/4 cup parsley, chopped
2 tsp dulse flakes
2 medjool dates, soaked in water for 1 hour
1 heaping tsp yellow mustard

Add all ingredients (except the cucumbers) to a food
processor and process until thoroughly combined.
Cut the cucumbers into slices.
Top each cucumber slice with a generous amount of tuno
salad.
Serve and enjoy!
Store leftover tuno salad in a glass container in the fridge for
up to 5 days.

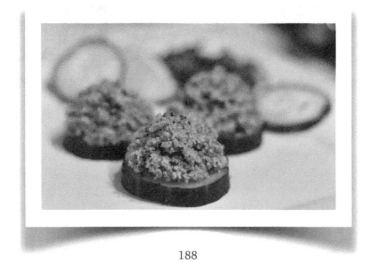

Veggie Loaf
Makes 3 servings

Loaf:
4 medium carrots, chopped
3 large stalks celery, chopped
2 cups frozen green peas, thawed
8 medium button mushrooms, chopped
1 cup sun-dried tomatoes, soaked in water for 20 minutes
then drained
1 cup sweet onion, chopped
2 garlic cloves, pressed or finely chopped
1/2 cup walnuts, soaked in water for 4 - 8 hours then rinsed
2 tsp paprika
2 tsp cumin
2 Tbsp chia seeds, ground
1 batch of Raw Ketchup

Raw Ketchup:
1 ½ cups grape tomatoes or 5 Roma tomatoes
1/2 cup sun-dried tomatoes, soaked in water for 1 hour
3 Medjool dates, pitted
2 tsp onion granules
2 Tbsp apple cider vinegar

Add all ingredients to a blender and blend until smooth.
Set Raw Ketchup to the side for now.

Add 2 Tbsp chia seeds to a high-speed blender or coffee
grinder and grind into powder.
Add all ingredients (except ketchup) to a food processor and
process until mixed well.
Place the processed mixture onto a dehydrator tray with a
teflex sheet and split into 3 equal parts.
Form the 3 portions of mixture into about 1-inch thick loaves.

Dehydrate at 105 degrees for 3 hours.

After 3 hours, remove the tray from the dehydrator and place another dehydrator tray without the teflex sheet on top of your 3 loaves, essentially sandwiching the loaves between the two dehydrator trays. Now, quickly but carefully flip the two trays over and remove the top tray along with the teflex sheet. The loaves will now be bottom up.

Place the tray with the loaves back into the dehydrator for 2 ½ hours.

Remove the tray from the dehydrator and apply a thin layer of ketchup on top of each loaf.

Place back into the dehydrator for 30 minutes.

Remove the loaves from the dehydrator, serve, and enjoy. Store leftovers in a glass container in the fridge for up to 5 days.

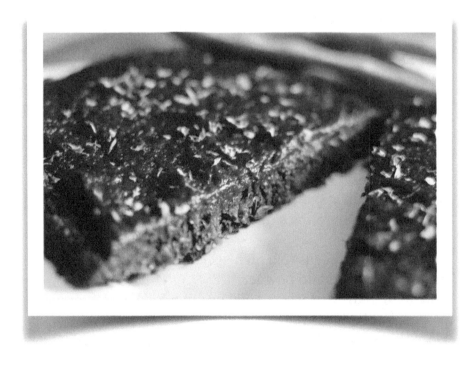

Wild Rice Stuffing
Makes 3 large servings

2 cups bloomed wild rice
1/2 cup soaked almonds
2 carrots
2 stalks celery
1/3 cup sweet onion
1 Tbsp lemon juice
2 tsp dried sage
2 tsp dried oregano
2 tsp dried thyme
1/4 cup fresh parsley, chopped
1 tsp apple cider vinegar or an additional 1 Tbsp lemon juice
1/4 cup water

Soak at least one cup of wild rice in 4 cups of clean water for 24 to 36 hours. This will give you about 2 cups of bloomed wild rice.
**To help your wild rice bloom better, you can run it through the food processor with the "S-blade" for about 1 minute before soaking. This puts small cuts in the outer layer of the rice and allows water to get inside easier to help it bloom.
Test the wild rice to make sure it has become soft and chewy. Many of the seeds should have broken open, showing the white inner portion.
When ready, drain the wild rice well and add two cups into a large mixing bowl and set to the side.
Place the almonds in a food processor and process with the S-blade until finely chopped.
Add the chopped almonds to your mixing bowl.
One at a time, in the food processor with the S-blade, finely chop the carrots, celery, onions, and parsley.
Add everything to the mixing bowl as you finish chopping each ingredient.

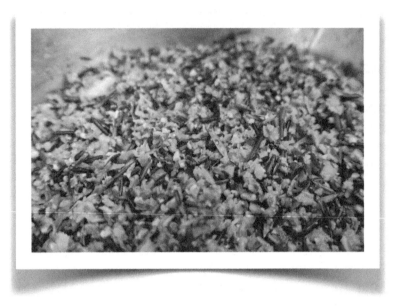

With a knife or in the food processor, finely chop the fresh parsley and add into the mixing bowl.

Add the sage, oregano, thyme, apple cider vinegar (or lemon juice), and water to the mixing bowl.

Mix everything very well.

Serve and enjoy.

Store leftovers in a glass container in the fridge for up to 5 days.

Zettuccine Alfredo and Meatless Balls
Makes 3 servings

Components:
5 large zucchini
1 cup of Hemp Garlic Sauce
3 Tbsp Raw Walnut Meat

Making the Zettucine Noodles:
Use a spiralizer or a julienne peeler to turn your 5 zucchini into noodles - peel the skin from the zucchini before spiralizing.

Place your zettucine noodles in a mixing bowl.

Hemp Garlic Sauce:
1/3 cup hemp seeds
1 cup peeled zucchini, chopped
1 clove garlic
1/4 cup yellow onion
3 Tbsp nutritional yeast
1 heaping tsp black pepper
1 tsp organic miso or 1 tsp sea salt
1 tsp psyllium husk powder
1 cup distilled water

Add all ingredients to a blender and blend until smooth.
Add 1 cup of Hemp Garlic Sauce to the mixing bowl.

Raw Walnut Meat:
3/4 cup walnuts, soaked in water for 4 - 8 hours then rinsed
3/4 cup sunflower seeds, soaked in water for 4 - 8 hours then rinsed
3/4 cup sun-dried tomatoes, soaked in water for 1 hour
1 cup sweet onion, chopped
1/2 cup parsley, chopped
2 tsp thyme
2 tsp sage
2 tsp paprika
2 tsp chili powder
1 clove garlic

Place all ingredients (except the chopped parsley) into a food processor with the "s-blade" and process until thoroughly combined.
Add the chopped parsley and pulse until it is well combined with the rest of the mixture.
Add 1 - 3 Tbsp of Walnut Meat to the mixing bowl.

Mix well until everything is thoroughly combined.
Serve and enjoy!

If desired, place the final mixture in a dehydrator set at 105 degrees Fahrenheit for 1 - 2 hours to soften the noodles and give it a more traditional pasta mouth-feel. You can also omit the Raw Walnut Meat for a fat free version of this recipe.

Store leftovers in glass containers in the fridge for up to 5 days.

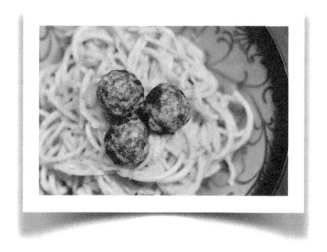

Zughetti and Meatless Balls
Makes 3 servings

Components:
5 large zucchini
1 cup of Raw Marinara Sauce
3 Tbsp Raw Walnut Meat
2 - 3 button mushrooms, thinly sliced and chopped

Making the Zughetti Noodles:

Use a spiralizer or a julienne peeler to turn your 5 zucchini into noodles - peel the skin from the zucchini before spiralizing.
Place your zughetti noodles in a mixing bowl.

Raw Marinara Sauce:
1 ½ cups grape tomatoes or 5 Roma tomatoes
1/2 cup sun-dried tomatoes, soaked in water for 1 hour
3 Medjool dates, pitted
2 tsp onion granules
2 Tbsp apple cider vinegar
2 Tbsp Frontier Pizza Seasoning

Add all ingredients to a blender and blend until smooth.
Add 1 cup of Marinara Sauce to the mixing bowl.

Raw Walnut Meat:
3/4 cup walnuts, soaked in water for 4 - 8 hours then rinsed
3/4 cup sunflower seeds, soaked in water for 4 - 8 hours
3/4 cup sun-dried tomatoes, soaked in water for at least 1 hour then rinsed
1 cup sweet onion, chopped
1/2 cup parsley, chopped
2 tsp thyme
2 tsp sage
2 tsp paprika
2 tsp chili powder
1 clove garlic

Place all ingredients (except the chopped parsley) into a food processor with the "s-blade" and process until thoroughly combined.
Add the chopped parsley and pulse until it is well combined with the rest of the mixture.
Add 1 - 3 Tbsp of Walnut Meat to the mixing bowl.

Add the thinly sliced and chopped mushrooms.

Mix well until everything is thoroughly combined.
Serve and enjoy!

If desired, place the final mixture in a dehydrator set at 105 degrees Fahrenheit for 1 - 2 hours to soften the noodles and give it a more traditional pasta mouth-feel. You can also omit the Raw Walnut Meat for a fat free version of this recipe.

Store leftovers in glass containers in the fridge for up to 5 days.

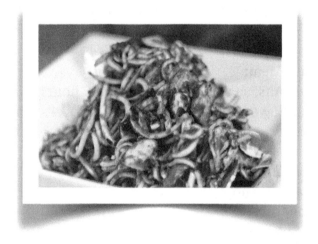

Smoothies

Banana Mango Bash
5 - 10 ripe bananas
1 - 2 cups frozen mango
1 - 2 cups spinach
1 - 2 tsp chia, flax, or hemp seeds (optional)
1 - 2 cups purified water, or to desired consistency

Add all of the ingredients into your blender.
Blend until smooth.

Berry Celebration
5 - 10 ripe bananas
1 - 2 cups frozen blueberries
2 stalks celery
2 - 3 Medjool dates
1 - 2 tsp chia, flax, or hemp seeds (optional)
1 - 2 cups purified water, or to desired consistency

Add all of the ingredients into your blender.
Blend until smooth.

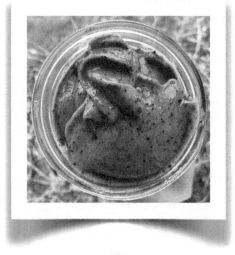

Berry Chocolate Dream

5 - 10 ripe bananas
2 - 3 Medjool dates
1 - 2 cups frozen blueberries
2 tsp carob powder
1 - 2 tsp chia, flax, or hemp seeds (optional)
1 - 2 cups purified water, or to desired consistency

Add all of the ingredients into your blender.
Blend until smooth.

Blueberry Basil Elation

5 - 10 ripe bananas
1 - 2 cups frozen blueberries
1 cup kale, chopped
1/4 cup fresh basil
1 - 2 tsp chia, flax, or hemp seeds (optional)
1 - 2 cups purified water, or to desired consistency

Add all of the ingredients into your blender.
Blend until smooth.

Blueberry Kale Infusion

5 - 10 ripe bananas
1 - 2 cups frozen blueberries
2 - 3 Medjool dates
1 cup kale
1 - 2 tsp chia, flax, or hemp seeds (optional)
1 - 2 cups purified water, or to desired consistency

Add all of the ingredients into your blender.
Blend until smooth.

Blueberry Mango Gratification

5 - 10 ripe bananas
1 cup frozen blueberries
1 cup frozen mango
1/4 cup cilantro
1 - 2 tsp chia, flax, or hemp seeds (optional)
1 - 2 cups purified water, or to desired consistency

Add all of the ingredients into your blender.
Blend until smooth.

Carob Berry Pie

5 - 10 ripe bananas
1 - 2 cups frozen strawberries
2 - 3 Medjool dates
1 Tbsp carob powder
1 - 2 tsp chia, flax, or hemp seeds (optional)
1 - 2 cups purified water, or to desired consistency

Add all of the ingredients into your blender.
Blend until smooth.

Cherry Berry Bonanza

5 - 10 ripe bananas
1 cup frozen cherries
1 cup frozen strawberries
1 cup arugula
1 - 2 tsp chia, flax, or hemp seeds (optional)
1 - 2 cups purified water, or to desired consistency

Add all of the ingredients into your blender.
Blend until smooth.

Cherry Maca Delight

5 - 10 ripe bananas
1 - 2 cups frozen cherries
2 tsp maca powder
1 - 2 tsp chia, flax, or hemp seeds
1 - 2 cups purified water, or to desired consistency

Add all of the ingredients into your blender.
Blend until smooth.

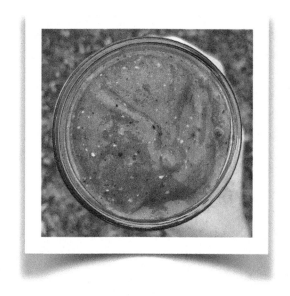

Cinnamon Sweet Surprise

5 - 10 ripe bananas
4 - 5 Medjool dates
1/4 tsp cinnamon
1 - 2 cups purified water (or to desired consistency)

Add all of the ingredients into your blender.
Blend until smooth.

Delectable Chocolate Shake

5 - 10 ripe bananas
3 - 4 Medjool dates
2 tsp carob powder
1 - 2 tsp chia, flax, or hemp seeds (optional)
1 - 2 cups purified water, or to desired consistency

Add all of the ingredients into your blender.
Blend until smooth.

Divine Sunrise

5 - 10 ripe bananas
1 cup frozen pineapple
1 - 2 navel oranges
1 cup spinach
1 - 2 tsp chia, flax, or hemp seeds (optional)
1 - 2 cups purified water, or to desired consistency

Add all of the ingredients into your blender.
Blend until smooth.

Hawaiian Green

5 - 10 ripe bananas
1 cup frozen pineapple
1 cup frozen mango
1 cup spinach
1 - 2 tsp chia, flax, or hemp seeds (optional)
1 - 2 cups purified water, or to desired consistency

Add all of the ingredients into your blender.
Blend until smooth.

Maca Mango Sunrise

5 - 10 ripe bananas
1 - 2 cups frozen mango

2 - 3 Medjool dates
2 tsp maca powder
1 - 2 tsp chia, flax, or hemp seeds (optional)
1 - 2 cups purified water, or to desired consistency

Add all of the ingredients into your blender.
Blend until smooth.

Pineapple Berry Awakening
5 - 10 ripe bananas
1 cup frozen pineapple
1 cup frozen strawberries
1 - 2 tsp chia, flax, or hemp seeds (optional)
1 - 2 cups purified water, or to desired consistency

Add all of the ingredients into your blender.
Blend until smooth.

Solar Burst
5 - 10 ripe bananas
1 - 2 cups frozen mango
1 - 2 navel oranges
1 - 2 cups kale
1 - 2 tsp chia, flax, or hemp seeds (optional)
1 - 2 cups purified water, or to desired consistency

Add all of the ingredients into your blender.
Blend until smooth.

Strawberry Basil Blast
5 - 10 ripe bananas
1 - 2 cups frozen strawberries
1/4 cup basil leaves
1 - 2 tsp chia, flax, or hemp seeds (optional)
1 - 2 cups purified water, or to desired consistency

Add all of the ingredients into your blender.
Blend until smooth.

Strawberry Mango Splash
5 - 10 ripe bananas
1 cup frozen strawberries
1 cup frozen mango
1 tsp chlorella powder
1 - 2 tsp chia, flax, or hemp seeds (optional)
1 - 2 cups purified water, or to desired consistency

Add all of the ingredients into your blender.
Blend until smooth.

Strawberry Shortcake
5 - 10 ripe bananas
1 - 2 cups strawberries
2 - 3 Medjool dates
2 tsp maca powder
1 - 2 tsp chia, flax, or hemp seeds (optional)
1 - 2 cups purified water, or to desired consistency

Add all of the ingredients into your blender.
Blend until smooth.

Sweet Detox
5 - 10 ripe bananas
1 - 2 cups frozen blueberries
2 - 3 Medjool dates
1/4 cup cilantro
1 tsp chlorella
1 - 2 tsp chia, flax, or hemp seeds (optional)
1 - 2 cups purified water, or to desired consistency

Add all of the ingredients into your blender.
Blend until smooth.

Tropical Celebration
5 - 10 ripe bananas
1 - 2 cups frozen mango
2 - 3 Medjool dates
2 stalks celery
1 - 2 tsp chia, flax, or hemp seeds (optional)
1 - 2 cups purified water, or to desired consistency

Add all of the ingredients into your blender.
Blend until smooth.

Dressings

Avocado Herb Dressing
1 medium hass avocado, mashed
1/2 lemon, juice only
2 tsp yellow mustard
1 Tbsp Kirkland's Organic No Salt Seasoning
Red pepper chili flakes to taste (optional)

Mix together until well combined.
Mix into your salad and enjoy!

Blazin' Cajun Dressing
3 Tbsp sunflower seeds
2 Medjool dates, pitted
1/2 lemon, peeled
1 clove garlic
1 tsp onion granules
1/2 tsp cajun seasoning
1/2 tsp paprika
1/4 tsp turmeric powder

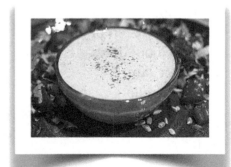

4 cup purified water

.dd all ingredients to a blender and blend until smooth. Pour over your salad and enjoy!

Brazilian Curry Dressing
3 Tbsp Brazil nuts
1 cloves garlic
2 Medjool dates, pitted
1/2 lemon, peeled
1 tsp curry powder
Pinch of cinnamon
1 tsp yellow mustard
1 cup purified water

Add all ingredients to a blender and blend until smooth. Pour over your salad and enjoy!

Brazilian Maca Dressing
3 Tbsp Brazil nuts (almonds can be substituted)
2 dates, pitted
1 clove garlic
1/2 lemon, peeled
1 heaping tsp Maca
1 tsp onion granules
1 cup purified water

Add all ingredients to a blender and blend until smooth.

Pour over your salad and enjoy!

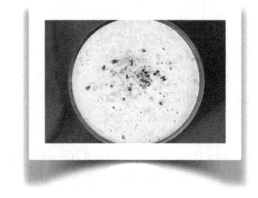

Buttermylk Dressing
3 Tbsp sesame seeds
3 medjool dates, pitted
1/2 lemon, peeled
1 Tbsp brown mustard
3/4 cup water

Add all ingredients to a blender and blend until smooth.
Pour over your salad and enjoy!

Cajun Red Dressing
3 Tbsp almonds
2 Medjool dates, pitted
1/2 lemon, peeled
1 tsp onion granules
1 tsp paprika
2 tsp Dijon mustard
1/2 tsp Cajun seasoning
3/4 cup water

Add all ingredients to a blender and blend until smooth,
Pour over your salad and enjoy!

Chili Brazily Dressing
3 Tbsp brazil nuts
2 medjool dates, pitted
1/2 lemon, peeled
1 tsp onion granules
1 tsp chili powder
1 tsp yellow mustard
1 cup purified water

Add all ingredients to a blender and blend until smooth.
Pour over your salad and enjoy!

hipotle Almond Dressing

Tbsp almonds
1/2 lemon, peeled
2 Medjool dates, pitted
1/2 tsp chipotle powder
1 tsp dijon mustard
3/4 cup purified water

Add all ingredients to a blender and blend until smooth.
Pour over your salad and enjoy!

Cowboy Sauce

3 Tbsp sesame seeds
1/3 cup red bell pepper
2 Medjool dates, pitted
1 clove garlic
1/2 lemon, peeled
1 tsp paprika
1/2 tsp red pepper flakes
3/4 cup water

Add all ingredients to a blender and blend until smooth.
Pour over your salad and enjoy!

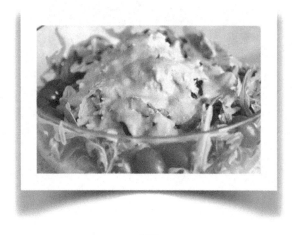

Creamy Italian Dressing

3 Tbsp sunflower seeds
1/2 lemon, peeled
2 Medjool dates, pitted
1 tsp onion granules
2 tsp Frontier Pizza Seasoning
3/4 cup purified water

Add all ingredients to a blender and blend until smooth.
Pour over your salad and enjoy!

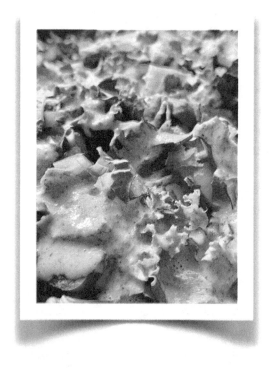

Illicious Dressing

Tbsp Sesame Seeds
1/2 lemon, peeled
2 Medjool dates, pitted
1 clove garlic
1 tsp onion granules
1 heaping tsp dijon mustard
1 heaping tsp dried dill
3/4 cup purified water

Add all ingredients to a blender and blend until smooth.
Pour over your salad and enjoy!

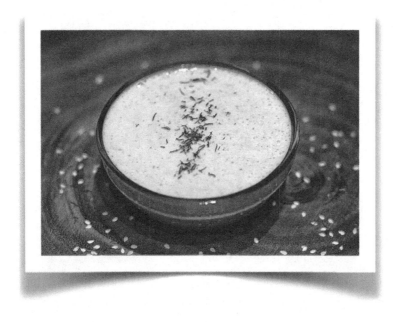

Rawnch Dressing
3 Tbsp hemp seeds
1 medium zucchini, peeled
1 tsp garlic granules
1 tsp onion granules
1 tsp dried dill
1 tsp chickpea miso
2 tsp chives, fresh or dried
1/2 lemon, peeled
1 tsp black pepper
1 tsp psyllium husk powder
3/4 cup purified water

Add all ingredients in a blender and blend until smooth. Pour on your salad and enjoy!

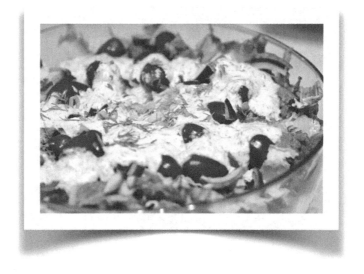

Royal Dragon Dressing
3 Tbsp sesame seeds
1/2 lemon, peeled
2 Medjool dates, pitted
2 tsp Dijon mustard

2 inch fresh ginger
clove garlic
tsp paprika
1/4 tsp cayenne pepper (or to taste)
3/4 cup water

Add all ingredients to a blender and blend until smooth. Pour over your salad and enjoy!

Sagemary Dressing
3 Tbsp sunflower seeds
1/2 lemon, peeled
2 Medjool dates, pitted
1 clove garlic
1 tsp onion granules
1 tsp dried rosemary
1 tsp dried sage
Pinch of cayenne pepper (to taste)
3/4 cup purified water

Add all ingredients to a blender and blend until smooth. Pour over your salad and enjoy!

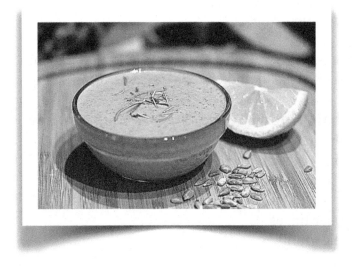

Sesame Sour Cream Dressing
3 Tbsp sesame seeds
2 Medjool dates, pitted
1/2 lemon, peeled
1 tsp garlic granules
1 tsp onion granules
1 tsp dijon mustard
1 Tbsp chives, fresh or dried
1 cup purified water

Add all ingredients (except the chives) to a blender and blend until smooth.
Add the chives and pulse until mixed well.
Pour over your salad and enjoy!

Smokehouse Dressing
3 Tbsp sunflower seeds
2 Medjool dates, pitted
1/2 lemon, peeled
1 clove garlic
1 tsp dijon mustard
1/2 tsp chili pepper flakes
1 tsp smoked paprika
3/4 cup purified water

Add all ingredients to a blender and blend until smooth.
Pour over your salad and enjoy!

Spicy Thai Almond Sauce
3 Tbsp almonds
1/2 lemon
1/4 inch ginger
2 dates
1 tsp pepper flakes
1 tsp garlic granules

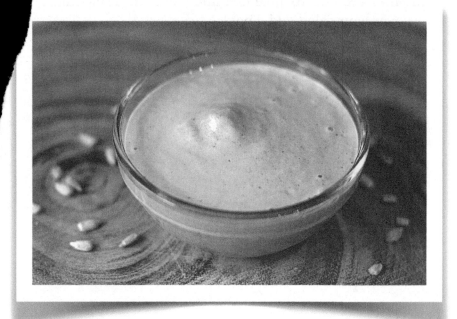

1 tsp organic miso
1/4 tsp paprika
3/4 cup water

Add all ingredients to a blender and blend until smooth.
Pour over your salad and enjoy!

Sunshine Curry Dressing
3 Tbsp sesame seeds
1/2 lemon, peeled
3 Medjool dates, pitted
2 tsp curry powder
1 tsp onion granules
1/4 tsp black pepper (or to taste)
1/2 jalapeno, chopped (remove seeds, if desired)
3/4 cup purified water

Add all ingredients to a blender and blend until smooth. Pour over your salad and enjoy!

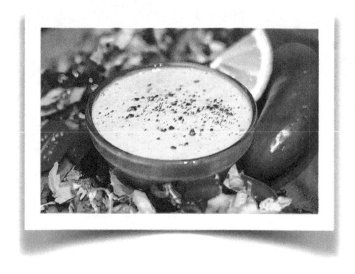

Sweet Masala Dressing
3 Tbsp sesame seeds
1/3 cup red bell pepper, chopped
2 medjool dates, pitted
1/2 lemon, peeled
1 tsp onion granules
2 tsp Frontier Tandoori Masala seasoning
1/4 tsp black pepper
1 pinch cayenne pepper
3/4 cup purified water

Add all ingredients to a blender and blend until smooth. Pour over your salad and enjoy!

Taco Supreme Dressing
3 Tbsp white sesame seeds
2 Medjool dates
1/4 cup red bell pepper

clove garlic

/2 lemon, peeled

 tsp Frontier taco seasoning

1/2 tsp paprika

1/8 tsp cayenne

3/4 cup purified water

Add all ingredients to a blender and blend until smooth.
Pour over your salad and enjoy!

Salads

Avocado, Corn, and Herb Salad
10 oz spinach, chopped
1 - 2 cups kale, finely chopped
1/4 cup cilantro, chopped
1/4 cup red onion, chopped
1/2 cucumber, chopped
1/2 to 1 cup frozen organic corn, thawed
2 carrots, shredded or chopped
7 - 10 grape tomatoes, whole or sliced

Add all ingredients to a large salad bowl and mix well.

Blazin' Cajun Salad
1/2 large head green leaf lettuce, chopped
2 cups spinach, chopped
1 cup kale, finely chopped
1/4 cup basil, chopped
1/3 cup red bell pepper, chopped
1/4 cup red onion, chopped
2 carrots, shredded or chopped
7 - 10 grape tomatoes, whole or sliced

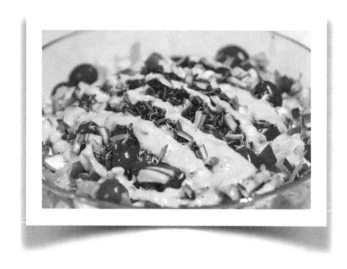

Add all ingredients to a large salad bowl and mix well.

Brazilian Curry Salad
1 large head green leaf lettuce, chopped
1 - 2 cups bok choy, chopped
1/4 cup dill, chopped
1/4 cup red onion, chopped
2 carrots, shredded or chopped
1/2 to 1 cup frozen peas, thawed
1/2 cucumber, chopped
7 - 10 grape tomatoes, whole or sliced

Add all ingredients to a large salad bowl and mix well.

Brazilian Maca Salad
1 medium to large head romaine lettuce, chopped
1 - 2 cups kale, finely chopped
1/4 cup cilantro, chopped
2 carrots, shredded or chopped
1/4 cup red onion, chopped
1/2 - 1 cup frozen green peas, thawed
7 - 10 grape tomatoes, whole or sliced

Add all ingredients to a large salad bowl and mix well.

ıttermylk Salad

1 large head romaine lettuce, chopped
1 - 2 cups kale, finely chopped
1/4 cup dill, chopped
1/4 cup red onion, chopped
2 stalks celery, chopped
2 carrots, shredded or chopped
7 - 10 grape tomatoes, whole or sliced

Add all ingredients to a large salad bowl and mix well.

Cajun Red Salad

1 large head green leaf lettuce, chopped
1 - 2 cups kale, chopped
1/4 cup cilantro, chopped
1/4 cup red onion, chopped
1/2 cucumber, chopped
2 carrots, chopped
7 - 10 grape tomatoes, whole or sliced

Add all ingredients to a large salad bowl and mix well.

Chili Brazily Salad

1 large head red leaf lettuce, chopped
1 - 2 cups arugula, chopped
1/4 cup parsley, chopped
1/4 cup yellow onion, chopped
1/2 cucumber, sliced or chopped
1/2 to 1 cup frozen green peas, thawed
1/2 cup button mushrooms, chopped
2 carrots, chopped
7 - 10 grape tomatoes, whole or sliced

Add all ingredients to a large salad bowl and mix well.

Chipotle Almond Salad
1/2 large head iceberg lettuce, chopped
1 cup red cabbage, shredded
1/4 cup basil, chopped
1/4 cup yellow onion, chopped
1/2 cucumber, chopped
1/2 - 1 cup frozen corn, thawed
2 carrots, shredded or chopped
7 - 10 grape tomatoes, whole or sliced

Add all ingredients to a large salad bowl and mix well.

Cowboy Salad
1 large head green leaf lettuce, chopped
1 - 2 cups bok choy, chopped
1/4 cup cilantro, chopped
1/4 cup red onion, chopped
1/2 to 1 cup frozen green peas, thawed
1/2 cucumber, chopped
2 carrots, chopped
7 - 10 grape tomatoes, whole or sliced

Add all ingredients to a large salad bowl and mix well.

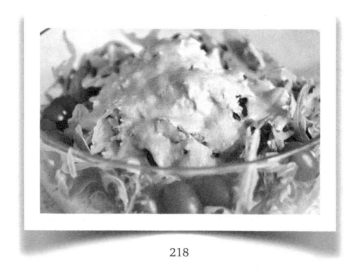

reamy Italian Salad
medium to large head green leaf lettuce, chopped
- 2 cups kale, finely chopped
1/4 cup basil, chopped
1/4 cup red onion, chopped
2 carrots, shredded or chopped
1/2 medium cucumber, chopped
7 - 10 grape tomatoes, whole or sliced

Add all ingredients to a large salad bowl and mix well.

Dillicious Salad
1/2 medium to large head green leaf lettuce, chopped
2 cups spinach, chopped
1 cup kale, finely chopped
1/4 cup cilantro, chopped
1/2 cucumber, chopped
1/4 cup red onion, chopped
1/2 - 1 cup frozen peas, thawed
2 carrots, shredded or chopped
7 - 10 grape tomatoes, whole or sliced

Add all ingredients to a large salad bowl and mix well.

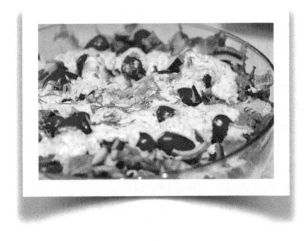

Rawnch Salad

1 large head romaine lettuce, chopped
1 - 2 cups bok choy, chopped
1/4 cup dill, chopped
1/4 cup red onion, chopped
2 stalks celery, chopped
1/2 to 1 cup frozen green peas, thawed
2 carrots, shredded or chopped
7 - 10 grape tomatoes, whole or sliced

Add all ingredients to a large salad bowl and mix well.

Royal Dragon Salad

1 large head romaine lettuce, chopped
1 - 2 cups bok choy, chopped
1/4 cup cilantro, chopped
1/4 cup red onion, chopped
1/3 cup celery, chopped
1/2 to 1 cup frozen peas, thawed
1/3 cup button mushrooms, chopped or sliced
2 carrots, shredded or chopped
7 - 10 grape tomatoes, whole or sliced

Add all ingredients to a large salad bowl and mix well.

Sagemary Salad

1/2 large head iceberg lettuce, chopped
1 - 2 cups arugula, chopped
1/4 cup parsley, chopped
1/4 cup yellow onion, chopped
1/3 beet, shredded
1/2 cucumber, chopped
2 carrots, shredded or chopped
7 - 10 grape tomatoes, whole or sliced
Add all ingredients to a large salad bowl and mix well.

esame Sour Cream Salad

/2 large head iceberg lettuce, chopped

- 2 cups arugula, chopped

1/4 cup parsley, chopped

1/4 cup yellow onion, chopped

1/2 to 1 cup frozen green peas, thawed

1/3 cup beet, shredded

2 carrots, shredded or chopped

7 - 10 grape tomatoes, whole or sliced

Add all ingredients to a large salad bowl and mix well.

Smokehouse Salad

1 medium to large head of romaine lettuce, chopped

1 - 2 cups kale, finely chopped

1/4 cup cilantro, chopped

2 carrots, shredded or chopped cup red onion, chopped

7 - 10 grape tomatoes, whole or sliced

2 stalks celery, chopped

Add all ingredients to a large salad bowl and mix well.

Spicy Thai Almond Salad

1 medium to large head of romaine lettuce, chopped

1 - 2 cups kale, finely chopped

1/4 cup cilantro, chopped

1/4 cup red onion, chopped

1/2 cup frozen corn, thawed

2 carrots, shredded or chopped

7 - 10 grape tomatoes, whole or sliced

Add all ingredients to a large salad bowl and mix well.

Sunshine Curry Salad
1/2 large head iceberg lettuce, chopped
1 cup red cabbage, shredded
1/4 cup basil, chopped
1/4 cup yellow onion, chopped
1/2 to 1 cup frozen corn, thawed
1/3 cup beet, shredded
2 stalks celery, chopped
7 - 10 grape tomatoes, whole or sliced

Add all ingredients to a large salad bowl and mix well.

Supreme Taco Salad
1 medium to large green leaf lettuce, chopped
1 - 2 cups kale, chopped
1/2 - 1 cup button mushrooms, chopped or sliced
1/2 cup frozen corn, thawed
1/4 cup red onion, chopped
1/3 cup red bell pepper, chopped
1/4 cup cilantro, chopped
2 carrots, shredded or chopped
7 - 10 grape tomatoes, whole or sliced

Add all ingredients to a large salad bowl and mix well.

Sweet Masala Salad
1 large head of red leaf lettuce, chopped
1 cup red cabbage, shredded
1/4 cup parsley, chopped
1/4 cup yellow onion, chopped
2 carrots, shredded or chopped
1/2 cucumber, chopped
7 - 10 grape tomatoes, whole or sliced

Add all ingredients to a large salad bowl and mix well.

About the Author:
Matt Bennett

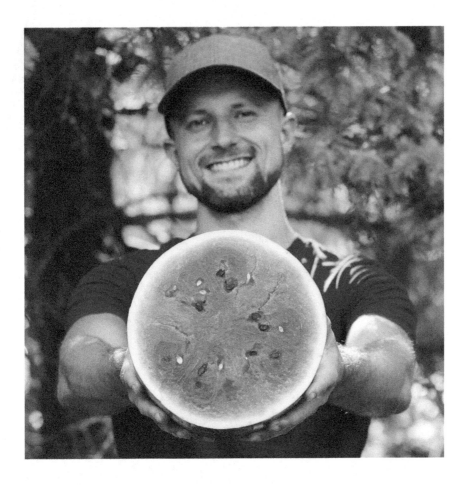

Matt Bennett is a Holistic Health Educator with a passionate focus on raw, living foods, and detoxification. Matt has been living a raw vegan lifestyle since 2011, and has experienced the healing of many of his childhood health conditions throughout that time. He now enjoys inspiring people to eat more raw fruits and vegetables with his educational ebooks, recipe ebooks, social media, and his monthly newsletter at myrawintuition.com.

Made in the USA
Las Vegas, NV
01 August 2024

93232712R00128